Management Essentials
for Doctors

Management Essentials for Doctors

Professor Rory Shaw
Medical Director
North West London Hospitals NHS Trust, London, UK
Senior Research Fellow, Imperial College, London, UK

Dr Vino Ramachandra
Consultant Anaesthetist
Northwick Park & St Mark's Hospitals, Harrow, UK

Dr Nuala Lucas
Consultant Anaesthetist
Northwick Park & St Mark's Hospitals, Harrow, UK

Dr Neville Robinson
Consultant Anaesthetist
Northwick Park & St Mark's Hospitals, Harrow, UK

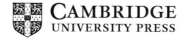
CAMBRIDGE
UNIVERSITY PRESS

CAMBRIDGE UNIVERSITY PRESS
Cambridge, New York, Melbourne, Madrid, Cape Town,
Singapore, São Paulo, Delhi, Tokyo, Mexico City

Cambridge University Press
The Edinburgh Building, Cambridge CB2 8RU, UK

Published in the United States of America
by Cambridge University Press, New York

www.cambridge.org
Information on this title: www.cambridge.org/9780521176798

First published 2011

Printed in the United Kingdom at the University Press, Cambridge

A catalogue record for this publication is available from the British Library

Library of Congress Cataloging in Publication data

Management essentials for doctors / Rory Shaw ... [et al.].
    p. ; cm.
  ISBN 978-0-521-17679-8 (Paperback)
  1. Great Britain. National Health Service.   2. Medical offices–Great
Britain–Management.   3. National health insurance–Great Britain.
I. Shaw, Rory.   II. Title.
  [DNLM: 1. Great Britain. National Health Service.   2. Practice
Management, Medical–organization & administration–Great Britain.
3. National Health Programs–organization & administration–Great
Britain. W 80]
  RA395.G7.M36 2011
  362.1068–dc22

                                                                2011012439

ISBN 978-0-521-17679-8 Paperback

Contents

Contributors

Mr Simon Lewis
Research Governance Manager
North West London Hospitals NHS Trust
UK

Dr Shriti Pattani
Occupational Health Consultant
North West London Hospitals NHS Trust
UK

Dr Alan Warnes
Research & Development Manager
North West London Hospitals NHS Trust
UK

Foreword

Professor Jenny Simpson OBE

For many years the mystique, magic and myths of healthcare management have presented a major challenge to doctors seeking to play a role in running the service. Even the terminology can be difficult to penetrate. Whilst there are many thousands of books detailing the intricacies of leadership and management, finding a source of information on who does what, why and where in the NHS can be a much greater challenge.

The journey through a doctor's clinical education can occasionally be haphazard, but compared with the totally random nature of a doctor's management development, however, it is a beautifully and consistently orchestrated process. No matter how enthusiastic a clinician may be to contribute to the management decision-making process, unless he or she happens to encounter a colleague with the insight and patience to show them around the basic anatomy, physiology and pathology of the NHS and the wider healthcare system, they will face many a difficulty in getting to grips with management. *Management Essentials for Doctors* fills this large gap, in that it provides a comprehensive guide to the full range of management functions and structures that can be so confounding.

Perhaps one of the most compelling reasons for having a copy of this book on the bookshelf is that it provides the answer to the questions that we might feel we should know the answer – but don't... *Management Essentials for Doctors* equips the reader to consider the complexities of healthcare management and ask sensible questions without being blocked by a lack of understanding of either the structures or the words. Whilst the theory of management in healthcare, with elegant analysis of the economics and organizational dynamics are well described elsewhere, this practical guide to the hugely complex and confounding pieces of the NHS jigsaw, how they fit together and how they are changing, is essential reading for clinicians trying to make sense of the environments in which they are likely to spend their entire working lives.

Covering all angles, from what the various medical management and leadership roles actually mean in terms of what people do, to the key issues of patient safety, clinical governance and performance management, this book is a 'must-have' for all doctors in training, those approaching an interview for a senior job – and for many an established GP and consultant as well.

Twenty years on from the beginnings of medical management in the UK, there is now no legitimacy for doctors to ignore their responsibilities as leaders and managers of clinical services. That battle was fought and won many years ago. In today's NHS, doctors will need to deliver their management and leadership roles with skill and confidence. *Management Essentials for Doctors* provides an ideal platform from which to pursue this ideal.

Preface

The doctor's frequent role as head of the healthcare team and commander of considerable clinical resource requires that greater attention is paid to management and leadership skills regardless of specialism.

Aspiring to Excellence, Professor Sir John Tooke, 2008

Management knowledge and skills are essential requirements for doctors of all grades. An understanding of all aspects of management is necessary for a doctor to perform at the highest standard. This book has been written by practising doctors for doctors. We have written the text with the aim of providing essential knowledge in a concise manner. We have included 60 topics in an easy-to-read format. The main themes have been alphabetically listed for easy reference. We have particularly focused on the 'nuts and bolts' of medical management, as these are the practical issues which impact on the daily lives of all doctors. Busy clinicians of all grades, educational leads and those taking up medical managerial roles will find this book particularly useful. Doctors preparing for interviews will also find that it provides the required knowledge for those management questions. We hope that our aims are met and that doctors will benefit from this book.

Rory Shaw
Vino Ramachandra
Nuala Lucas
Neville Robinson

Acknowledgements

In the course of creating this book we have drawn on the time and support of many people. Our colleagues in R&D, Dr Alan Warnes and Mr Simon Lewis, wrote chapters on 'Research funding' and 'Research governance', respectively; Dr Shriti Pattani, Consultant in Occupational Health, contributed a chapter on 'The sick doctor'. We thank them for giving of their time generously and keeping to deadlines. We are also grateful to Ms Fiona Wise, chief executive, North West London Hospitals NHS Trust, for her support; consultant colleagues for their encouragement and helpful suggestions; our trainees for inspiring us to write this book; and Deborah Russell and Jane Seakins at Cambridge University Press for having been a constant source of help throughout its preparation.

Last, but not least, a special thanks to our loving, supportive and understanding families.

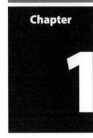

Chapter

Audit

There are various definitions available for audit but one of the most common is 'a quality improvement process that seeks to improve patient care and outcomes through systematic review of care against explicit criteria and the implementation of change'. Audit is so ubiquitous in healthcare that it is easy to forget that it is a relatively new innovation. The concept for audit was first mooted in the 1970s. With the publication of the 1989 White Paper 'Working for Patients: Medical Audit Working Paper No. 6', detailed plans for a comprehensive system of medical audit within the internal market were proposed. A massive drive to develop medical audit began. Protected funding was made available to support it. With the advent of clinical governance in the mid 1990s, audit is now firmly established as an integral part of healthcare delivery.

Audit can encompass managerial and financial components of the healthcare delivery process, but the most relevant to clinicians is clinical audit. Clinical audit is essentially a checking process to assess the quality and effectiveness of any aspect of healthcare delivery and making change or improvements where necessary. It is usually described as an audit cycle. The audit cycle encompasses identifying a clinical area or objective to be audited, agreeing the standard or benchmark for the audit (minimum level of acceptable performance), data collection that describes or measures current performance, analysing the results and identifying the areas for change or improvement and, lastly, re-auditing after the change has been implemented. Clinical audit can be retrospective or prospective. Retrospective audit is probably of most use in the event of critical incident (serious untoward incident resulting in severe morbidity or death) or when a complaint or litigation has arisen and a review of practice is required urgently. In the development of any clinical audit programme retrospective audit may have a role but, for audit to contribute meaningfully to improving quality of care, the majority of clinical audit should be prospective. Prospective clinical audit allows for accurate contemporaneous collection of data reflecting current rather than historical practice. Data is therefore more likely to be accurate in volume and detail.

Participation in clinical audit is a mandatory requirement for doctors at all levels. General Medical Council (GMC) recommendations are that all doctors 'must take part in regular and systematic audit' and that individual doctors must 'respond constructively to the outcome of audit' (General Medical Council, 2006).

Advantages of audit

As well as improving the quality of healthcare, clinical audit has other potential benefits:

- Improved multidisciplinary team working
- Improved working environment and greater openness to change

- Provides reassurance to patients and clinical staff that best practice standards are being met
- Can assist with the development of local guidelines or protocols
- Can reduce incidents, complaints and claims.

Choice of clinical audit

The choice of clinical audit should reflect national topics. Recommendations come from the Department of Health and the National Institute for Health and Clinical Excellence (NICE). Many of the Royal Colleges also provide advice on areas that should be audited and in some instances a selection of 'audit recipes' to facilitate audit. In addition, the choice of topics should be based on the traditional criteria of:

- High volume: frequent procedures or many patients or users involved
- High risk: the procedure or intervention may lead to harm to patients or users, staff or the organization
- High profile: causes of concern have already been identified, e.g. complaints and quality incidents
- High cost: activities that are costly in monetary terms or resources.

Clinical audit is a multidisciplinary process and therefore selection of topics should also look at those areas that can maximize the involvement of as many members of the teams delivering care as possible. Other factors that should be considered include:

- Is it practical to undertake the audit and who needs to be involved?
- Is the problem amenable to change?
- Is the subject a priority for the hospital, practice or service?
- Are national standards or recommendations available against which to benchmark?

The re-invigoration of clinical audit

Since 2006, following the Chief Medical Officer's report 'Good Doctors, Safer Patients', there has been a national drive to re-invigorate clinical audit. There are three main groups involved in this drive:

- NICE
- National Clinical Audit Advisory Group (NCAAG): established by the Department of Health to drive the re-invigoration programme and provide a national focus for discussion and advice on matters relating to clinical audit
- Healthcare Quality Improvement Partnership (HQIP): established in April 2008 to promote quality in healthcare, and in particular to increase the impact that clinical audit has on healthcare quality in England and Wales. It is led by a consortium of the Academy of Medical Royal Colleges, the Royal College of Nursing and National Voices (a coalition of national health and social care organizations).

HQIP has a contract with the Department of Health to manage and develop the National Clinical Audit and Patient Outcomes Programme (NCAPOP). This programme is a set of centrally funded national projects that use a common format to help individual trusts to collect audit data. The collected data is analysed centrally and trusts can then use this data to help identify necessary improvements for patients. A wide range of medical, surgical and mental health conditions is already included in this programme; most notably the Paediatric Intensive Care Audit Network (PICANet) and the National Joint Registry (NJR).

Reference and further reading

http://www.hqip.org.uk (accessed 6 January 2011).

GMC (2006). *Guidance for Doctors. Good Medical Practice*. London: GMC.

Care bundles

In 2004 the Modernisation Agency published '10 High Impact Changes for Service Improvement and Delivery'. By working with many clinical teams nationally, these 10 high impact changes for the delivery of healthcare were identified. The implementation of care bundles in the NHS was high impact change no. 6.

A 'care bundle' is a collection of interventions that, when implemented together, will achieve significantly better outcomes for patients, such as reduced mortality and morbidity and improved cost-effectiveness. They are used in specific clinical situations and aim to improve the consistency with which healthcare is delivered.

The features of a care bundle are as follows:

- All steps are necessary and each step must be performed to achieve success
- Each step is evidence-based (usually level 1 evidence)
- A bundle should include 3–5 steps. The chances of the bundle being carried out in full and being successful reduce with every step that is added
- The bundle must be completed in the same time and place continuum
- Each step of the bundle should be clearcut, being completed in a yes/no fashion
- The care bundle should be easily accessible by clinicians.

These features make care bundles distinct from checklists and guidelines.

Benefits of care bundles

The benefits of using care bundles are not only confined to patient outcomes. There are also benefits in terms of the following:

- **Service delivery**
  - Improved clinical governance procedures
  - Improved equity of care between patients
  - Faster delivery of care because of explicit agreement on therapies
  - Possibility of decreased length of stay
  - Possibility of decreased cost.
- **Patient experience**
  - Fewer complications
  - Fewer complaints
  - Fewer omissions of indicated therapy
  - Reduction in unnecessary length of stay and other risks of hospitalization.

- **Clinical outcomes**
  - Reduced morbidity
  - Improved outcomes if therapy is given more regularly
  - Treatment is based on agreed, evidence-based guidelines
  - Fewer adverse events
  - Fewer complications as prophylaxis regimens are administered more regularly
  - Links between outcomes and processes more evident.
- **Benefits for staff**
  - Clinical and managerial staff aligned to provide the best care for patients
  - A systematic approach to improve the delivery of healthcare is encouraged
  - Creative discussion between staff leads to new insights on care processes
  - Improved relationships between staff by stimulating dialogue.

(Source: http://www.ogc.gov.uk/documents/Health_High_Impact_Changes.pdf (accessed 6 January 2011)).

The use of care bundles originated from work in intensive care units in the USA. The advent of the International Surviving Sepsis campaign further popularized their use. This was a joint collaboration between the European Society of Intensive Care Medicine, the International Sepsis Forum and the Society of Critical Care Medicine to improve care and reduce the numbers of deaths worldwide from sepsis; the management principles under-lying this campaign included care delivered as bundles. More recently a major UK study aimed to look at the use of care bundles outside of the intensive care setting (for diseases such as diarrhoea and vomiting, stroke, chronic obstructive pulmonary disease and heart failure). This study demonstrated a reduction in hospital standardized mortality rate consistent with other studies on the subject. The authors make the point that it is impossible to assume a causal relationship between introducing the targeted care bundles and the reduced mortality. However, the significant reduction in mortality occurred only at the site where the care bundles were predominantly used.

Further reading

Robb, E., Jarman, B., Suntharalingam, G. *et al.* (2010). Using care bundles to reduce in-hospital mortality: quantitative survey. *British Medical Journal*, **340**: c1234.

Checklists

In the past 10 years there has been a huge increase in interest in ways to improve patient safety and reduce iatrogenic injury. The development of checklists in medicine is one such way. In the USA in 1999 the Institute of Medicine (a non-governmental organization whose purpose is to provide national advice on issues relating to health and medicine) published 'To Err is Human: Building a Safer Health System'. This report looked at medical errors in the USA. This was followed in 2001 by 'Crossing the Quality Chasm', which investigated further elements of the 1999 report. These reports were the inspiration for the widely publicized '100,000 lives campaign' in the USA, aimed at reducing hospital morbidity and mortality in a number of key areas, e.g. the prevention of central line infections and surgical site infections.

Enthusiasm for checklists grew following the publication of the 'Michigan' or 'Keystone' paper. Peter Pronovost, an American intensivist at Johns Hopkins, devised a simple five-point checklist to accompany central line cannulation in an intensive care unit. He created the list after extensive literature review and he chose for the checklist the five points that were most likely to be effective in reducing line-associated infection. The checklist was therefore a standardized, evidenced-based tool. The use of the checklist was associated with a dramatic reduction in infection in the intensive care unit.

A checklist describes the key steps that must be carried out to ensure a procedure is completed safely. They can be procedure-specific for use by an individual, e.g. insertion of a central line, or process-specific for use by a team, e.g. the surgical safety checklist. They work by improving recall, and it has been suggested that the 'Hawthorne effect' (a tendency to perform better when an individual is being observed) may also play a part in their success.

The use of checklists in medicine has gathered momentum with the advent of the World Health Organization's second Global Patient Safety Challenge, 'Safe Surgery Saves Lives Campaign', launched in June 2008 to reduce the number of surgical deaths worldwide. The initiative has been led in the UK by the National Patient Safety Agency (NPSA). Probably the most widely used clinical checklist in the UK is the 'surgical safety checklist'. Since February 2010 it has been mandatory that a 'surgical safety checklist' be used for all surgical procedures. The aims of the surgical safety checklist include:

- Improved anaesthetic safety
- Reduced occurrence of wrong-site surgery
- Avoidance of surgical site infections
- Improved communication among the surgical team.

The surgical safety checklist comprises three components: sign in, to be completed before induction of anaesthesia; time out, completed before commencement of surgery; and sign out, completed before the patient leaves the operating theatre. Modified checklists, available on the NPSA website, have been produced specifically for radiological procedures, cataract surgery and obstetrics.

A study from the Netherlands recently published in the *New England Journal of Medicine* confirms that surgical safety checklists are effective in reducing surgical morbidity and mortality (de Vries *et al.*, 2010).

Checklists clearly have a role in improving patient safety; however, the provision of a simple tick box list is not enough; the use of checklists needs to be accompanied by a cultural change in that particular healthcare setting. Also, healthcare professionals need to be motivated to take part, e.g. when utilizing the surgical safety checklist any member of the theatre team can lead the checklist, and all members of the team need to feel empowered enough to challenge others. Audit is also an integral part of the process when using a checklist to ensure compliance and effectiveness.

Checklists may not be suitable for use in all aspects of medicine and even when they have proved to be useful in specific situations they may need to be modified in some circumstances, e.g. the use of a surgical safety checklist should not cause delay in emergency surgery.

Checklists clearly have an important role to play in patient safety but they are not a panacea. Peter Pronovost has warned of the risk of 'checklist overload', the creation of too many checklists, particularly if there is no clear benefit to patients. There is also the risk that checklists may lead to complacency and a false sense of security.

References and further reading

Bosk, C.L., Dixon-Woods, M., Goeschel, C.A. and Pronovost, P.J. (2009). Reality check for checklists. *Lancet*, **374**: 444–5.

De Vries, E.N., Prins, H.A., Crolla, R.M.P.H. *et al.* (2010). Effect of a comprehensive surgical safety system on patient outcomes. *New England Journal of Medicine*, **363**: 1928–37.

Haynes, A.B., Weiser, T.G., Berry, W.R. *et al.* (2009). A surgical safety checklist to reduce morbidity and mortality in a global population. (Safe Surgery Saves Lives Study Group.) *New England Journal of Medicine*, **360**: 491–9.

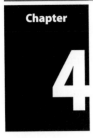

Core knowledge

Clinical dashboards

A clinical dashboard is a way of presenting information and data, and tracking changes about various aspects of healthcare delivery. The dashboard can be presented with visual displays, pie charts, etc., or simple Excel spreadsheets. The aims of using a dashboard are several: comparing local activity to national targets or standards, clinical governance and risk management.

The term dashboard comes from the analogy with the information provided on a car dashboard. On a car dashboard, red lights flash when there is cause for concern, so the clinical dashboard employs the same system. Thresholds are set using local or national figures where available. Areas where there is no cause for concern are marked as green, where action is required to improve or prevent further deterioration they are marked as amber, and areas that require urgent intervention are marked as red.

The idea evolved from its use in obstetrics, and it is now a Royal College of Obstetricians and Gynaecologists' (RCOG) recommendation. The RCOG suggest four categories where data may be collected:

- Clinical activity
- Workforce
- Clinical outcomes
- Risk incidents/complaints or patient satisfaction surveys.

The development of clinical dashboards was a key recommendation from both Lord Darzi's major review of the NHS ('Next Stage Review'), published in June 2008, and the Health Informatics Review, published in July 2008.

Stages of development of clinical dashboards

A prototype phase began in April 2008 and aimed to provide 'proof of concept'. Three NHS organizations worked with NHS Connecting for Health to develop the first clinical dashboard 'prototypes'. The organizations involved were:

- Nottingham University Hospital (Urology dashboard)
- Homerton University Foundation Trust (A&E dashboard)
- Bolton Primary Care Trust (PCT) (GP practice and primary care dashboard).

Following this, a pilot phase was implemented in November 2009, which aimed to evaluate the potential benefits of using a clinical dashboard within a broader range of clinical settings across the UK. Across the 10 strategic health authorities in England, 24 dashboards were developed in hospital-based settings, general practice and other community-based clinical teams. During this phase the core technical infrastructure necessary for implementation of dashboards was developed and collated into a 'toolkit' to facilitate a planned national roll-out.

Benefits of using a clinical dashboard

The pilot phase of development established that with well motivated local clinical leadership, dashboards can help staff to deliver accurate, contemporaneous information about healthcare delivery that can improve the quality of healthcare.

The benefits of using a clinical dashboard can be summarized as follows:

- Better information for clinical teams, presented in an easy-to-understand format with high visual impact
- Utilization of multiple sources of existing data, providing clinical information which is relevant across a multidisciplinary team
- Information provided in 'real time', facilitating immediate targeted decisions to improve patient care and avoiding delays by data cleansing processes
- Improved data quality through immediate, day-to-day visualization of data reinforces 'capture once, use many times' behaviours.

Challenges of a clinical dashboard

Clinical dashboards have proved to be an effective tool in the clinical governance process. However, the development of a clinical dashboard in any setting requires significant input to ensure the accuracy and quality of the information provided. The pilot project established that dashboards are not effective without clinical and executive level support or when data used to supply the dashboards was poor. Significant investment is required to achieve this. Therefore it has been suggested that each organization makes its own decision as to whether clinical dashboards are right for them and that, if they decide to proceed, local formal review is required to elucidate which clinical areas should be targeted.

Further reading

http://www.connectingforhealth.nhs.uk/
    systemsandservices/clindash/benefits
    (accessed 13 December 2010)

Core knowledge

Complaints procedure

A complaint can be defined as an expression of dissatisfaction requiring a response. Complaints are widespread in the health service. They can come from patients, relatives, carers or other healthcare workers.

The new shared complaints procedure for both health and social care came into force on 1 April 2009. It is structured around three main principles: listening, responding and improving. The premise for the reform was to give organizations the flexibility they need to deal with complaints more effectively and also encourage a culture that seeks and uses people's experiences to make services effective, personal and safe. This new complaints procedure represents a significant attempt to improve the management of patient, carer and public concerns in a complainant-centred manner.

The NHS Constitution

The NHS Constitution was published in January 2009 and states that every patient and carer has the right to:

- Have any complaint they make about NHS services dealt with efficiently and be properly investigated
- Know the outcome of any investigation into their complaint
- Take their complaint to the independent health service ombudsman if they are not satisfied with the way their complaint has been dealt with by the NHS
- Make a claim for judicial review if they think they have been directly affected by an unlawful act or decision by an NHS body
- Compensation where they have been harmed by negligent treatment.

The Health Act 2009 places a duty on NHS organizations to have regard to the NHS Constitution.

What do patients complain about?

Common reasons for complaints:

- Long waits: for appointments, investigations, therapies and operations
- Delays in treatment
- Cancellation of appointments and operations
- Poor or no communication
- Staff attitudes and bedside manners
- Environment: cleanliness, parking charges, food

- Clinical decisions
- Mistakes
- Harm.

What outcomes do patients seek?

In general, patients want improvements, disclosure of events and reassurances that lessons will be learnt, so that the same will not happen again. Less than 10% of complainants seek financial compensation.

Procedure for managing complaints

- Patients now have 12 months from the event occurrence or becoming aware of the event, to complain. This time period can be extended to allow for such things as the complainant grieving or undergoing other trauma or an anxiety state requiring treatment
- There are now only two stages to the complaints procedure: local resolution and recourse to the parliamentary and health service ombudsman. The Health Care Commission no longer plays a role
- Written, formal complaints must be acknowledged in writing within 3 working days of receipt. The complainant must be given the name and contact details of the investigating officer or designated complaints manager and offered an opportunity to meet the key staff involved
- It is important to go through the reasons for their unhappiness with the complainant systematically. Ask them what they would like to happen as a result of the complaint: an apology, explanation, improvements, reimbursement of costs, new appointment, legal action, compensation, etc.
- Complainants should be made aware of both the organization's Patient Advice and Liaison Services (PALS) and the Independent Complaints Advocacy Service (ICAS). PALS advise complainants how to take their complaint forward or resolve it informally. ICAS is a free, confidential and independent service which helps patients and carers make a formal complaint about NHS services
- Once a complaint has been fully investigated, the chief executive (secondary care) or responsible person (primary care) must send a response to the complainant. This response letter must include an apology (not necessarily accepting blame or fault), address each of the issues in turn and include details of the investigation and any action taken by the organization/practice. With cross-boundary complaints, the complainant must be given a coordinated response
- If legal action is implied or indicated or compensation sought, the matter should be passed on to legal services
- Complaints can be made to the GMC directly, especially if the complaint against a doctor is about conduct and performance issues.

Handling complaints is both time-consuming and stressful. If a complaint escalates, it can damage a doctor's reputation and lead to GMC referral and litigation. In primary care they can also damage relations with the primary care trust. It is important therefore to try and prevent the generation of a complaint by communicating with patients at the time of the incident or as soon as possible after the event. If dealt with promptly and sympathetically, it is often possible to resolve a complaint at an early stage without going through the formal complaints procedure. It is well recognized that when complaints are dealt with in an effective manner there is a reduction in legal recourse.

Retaining complaints

Complaint letters from patients must not be kept in their health record. Files need to be kept securely and information only shared on a need-to-know basis. In hospitals, files have to be retained for at least 10 years. Mental health, obstetrics and paediatric complaints must be retained for much longer periods. There is now a requirement that doctors retain records of complaints and their outcomes in their appraisal portfolios.

Steps to a good complaint response

- Apology – if there has been a failure to meet an expected standard
- Acknowledgement – recognition that things could have been better or different
- Action – give an assurance that as a result of the issues raised, practice has changed or schedules altered.

Dealing with serious complaints

Sometimes a complaint can raise serious safety issues for service users or the general public – for instance, a complaint alleging a serious failure in standards of care by an individual health or social care worker or a particular hospital service. In such cases it is essential that the complaints are investigated promptly as the safety of others depends on taking swift and effective action. Remember the following:

- A single incident may be a symptom of a more systematic problem in the performance or conduct of the individual or service about which the complaint is being made
- Conversely, a complaint about the conduct of an individual may turn out on closer investigation to relate to an underlying problem in the team or organization in which they work
- If the complaint relates to serious harm or a significant 'near miss', consider reporting it as a serious untoward incident
- Ensure that the investigation is fair and transparent with a sufficient degree of independence to be credible
- Ensure that the professional who is subject to the complaint has access to professional support and, if they wish, occupational health resources during and after the investigation.

Further reading

NHS Complaints Procedure: www.dh.gov.uk/en/Managingyourorganization (accessed 2 May 2010).

The Parliamentary and Health Service Ombudsman: www.ombudsman.org.uk (accessed 7 November 2010).

NHS Complaints in England: www.medicalprotection.org/uk/booklets/nhs-complaints-in-england (accessed 7 November 2010).

Patient Advice and Liaison Services: www.pals.nhs.uk (accessed 7 November 2010).

European Working Time Directive

The European Working Time Directive (EWTD) is a directive from the Council of European Union (93/104/EC) to protect the health and safety of workers in the European Union. It lays down minimum requirements in relation to working hours, rest periods, annual leave and working arrangements. The Directive was enacted in UK law and took effect from 1 October 1998. It has applied to both consultants and non-consultant career grades since implementation. However, doctors in training were exempted until August 2004, when a phased reduction from 58 hours to 48 hours in 2009 applied. The working time regulations place a legal requirement on employers and build on the progress made through the New Deal. Contracts requiring doctors in training to work outside the Regulations are now illegal.

Key aspects

- No more than 48 hours per week, averaged over a reference period
- 11 hours' continuous rest in 24 hours
- 24 hours continuous rest in 7 days (or 48 hours in 14 days)
- 20-minute break in work periods of over 6 hours
- 4 weeks' annual leave
- For night workers, an average of no more than 8 hours' work in 24 over the reference period.

For doctors in training the reference period is 26 weeks. This means that in some weeks it is possible that a doctor may work more than 48 hours. Doctors in training also have an individual right to opt out if they choose to do so, but they cannot opt out of rest break or leave requirements. There is some provision within the Directive to apply a variation by collective agreement. This is known as 'derogation'. In the case of junior doctors it is possible to derogate from the minimum daily rest requirements set out by the Working Time Directive (WTD). The UK has derogated from these terms, and junior doctors are entitled to a 'compensatory' rest equivalent to that which is lost when the ideal daily rate is not achieved.

SiMAP and Jaegar judgments

The SiMAP judgment refers to a case brought before the European Court of Justice on behalf of a group of Spanish doctors. The ruling declared that all time spent resident on-call would count as working time. Whilst the ruling applied to a specific case, the assumption is that if British doctors work under similar arrangements, then a similar interpretation of 'working time' applies. The European Court of Justice judgment on Jaegar followed the SiMAP line.

Working practices that could deliver compliance with the WTD

- Development of emergency medical teams providing cover across a hospital at night
- New non-medical roles supporting and substituting for doctors in training
- Reduction of number of tiers of emergency medical cover
- New service models
- New team-working patterns.

Summary of the Temple report 'Time for training: a review of the impact of the EWTD on the quality of training'

This review was commissioned by Medical Education England and looked at the impact of the EWTD on the quality and training of doctors, dentists, pharmacists and healthcare scientists. It was led by Professor Sir John Temple and the main findings and recommendations were as follows:

Findings

High quality training can be delivered within the 48-hour week, but this is precluded when trainees have a major role in out-of-hours services, are poorly supported and have limited access to learning. Gaps in rotas result in lost training opportunities, since trainees are then asked to increase the proportion of out-of-hours work that they do. The impact of the EWTD is greatest in specialties with high emergency and/or out-of-hours workloads. Traditional models of training and service delivery waste learning opportunities. The considerable increase in junior doctor numbers to meet EWTD has reinforced traditional patterns of working and diluted training opportunities. Consultant ways of working often support the traditional training models. Despite significant consultant expansion, trainees are still responsible for initiating and frequently delivering the majority of out-of-hours service, often with limited supervision. Service reconfiguration and redesign can provide a better, safer service to patients and enhance the quality of training. Where organizations have proactively designed new ways in which they work and train to meet all the changes affecting the service, a number of benefits have been identified:

- The expansion of consultant presence can result in efficiency savings and enhanced patient safety
- Splitting services into elective and emergency has enhanced training, delivered EWTD-compliant rotas and improved quality of care
- Hospital at Night allows trainees to maximize their daytime working while providing safe patient care at night
- Simulation and new technologies can support training and accelerate learning
- Multidisciplinary team-working can provide trainees with valuable training opportunities and reduce their workload
- Mentoring and support of newly appointed consultants enables them to be both competent and confident.

Recommendations

Implement a consultant-delivered service

Consultants must be more directly responsible for the delivery of 24/7 care. Consultants will need to work more flexibly to deliver high quality training and service. The roles of consultants need to be developed for them to be more directly involved in out-of-hours care. A clear alignment between service need and the number of new Certificate of Completion of Training (CCT) awards, in terms of workforce planning, is urgently needed to enable a consultant-delivered model. The doctors clinically responsible for service delivery should be employed in substantive posts under the consultant contract. An expansion of any other grade will not support a move to a consultant-delivered service model. Newly appointed consultants need mentoring and support. Training should be delivered in a service environment with appropriate, graded consultant supervision.

Service delivery must explicitly support training

Services must be designed and configured to deliver high quality patient care and training. This may be at a department, trust, regional or national level, depending on the local circumstances and specialty involved, but will require the necessary critical mass of professionals to maintain a viable service. As the ratio of trainees to consultants changes with increasing consultant numbers, it may no longer be feasible to train in all hospitals. Re-configuration or redesign of elective and emergency services and an effective Hospital at Night programme are two of the ways in which healthcare can be changed to support training and ensure safe services. Rotas require organization and effective management to maximize training in 48 hours. Current employment contracts need to be re-appraised to ensure that they support training within the EWTD. Multidisciplinary team-working must be used to support training.

Make every moment count

Training must be planned and focused for each trainee's needs. Trainers and trainees must use learning opportunities in every clinical situation. Handovers can be an effective learning experience when supervised by senior staff, preferably consultants. The coordinated, integrated use of simulation and technology can provide a safe, controlled environment to accelerate learning. Mentoring and support for trainees must be improved. Training requires a change from traditional perceptions of learning to a model which recognizes the modern NHS. Trainees must be involved in the decision-making and implementation of training innovations that affect their present and future careers. Extending the hours worked or the length of training programmes are not sustainable solutions.

Further reading

House, J. (2009). Calling time on doctors' working hours. *Lancet*, **373**(9680): 2011–12.

A guide to the implementation of the European Working Time Directive for doctors in training: www.dh.gov.uk (accessed 6 July 2010).

Time for training: a review of the impact of the EWTD on the quality of training (2010): www.mee.nhs.uk (accessed 6 July 2010).

Good medical practice

The 2006 GMC publication *Good Medical Practice* sets out the principles and values upon which good practice is founded and is the professional code of practice for doctors in the UK. The guidance is addressed to doctors, but it is also intended to let the public know what they can expect from doctors. The seven domains constitute the basis for satisfactory appraisal and assessment of all doctors. Every Royal College has used the guidance to formulate good practice guidelines specific to their specialty.

The seven domains are:

- Good clinical care
- Maintaining good medical practice
- Teaching and training, appraising and assessing
- Relationships with patients
- Working with colleagues
- Probity
- Health.

Each domain has several subsections as outlined below.

Good clinical care

- Providing good clinical care
- Supporting self-care
- Avoid treating those close to you
- Raising concerns about patient safety
- Decisions about access to medical care
- Treatment in emergencies.

The guidance emphasizes the need for: assessing patients adequately, heeding patients' views, arranging appropriate investigations and treatments based on best available evidence, recognizing and working within the limits of your competence, prescribing appropriately, keeping clear, accurate, legible and contemporaneous records, being readily available when on duty, respecting patients' rights to a second opinion, encouraging patients and the public to improve and maintain their health, treating patients without discrimination, avoiding treating close relations, and raising concerns about patient safety in the appropriate manner.

Maintaining good medical practice

- Keeping up to date
- Maintaining and improving your performance.

In this section there is a clear requirement for keeping knowledge and skills up to date throughout your working life as well as working with colleagues, patients and regulatory bodies to maintain and improve the quality of your work and promote patient safety.

Teaching and training, appraising and assessing

The guide emphasizes the need to ensure that all staff for whom you are responsible are properly supervised, and for being honest and objective when appraising and assessing the performance of colleagues, students and locums. If you are involved in teaching you must develop the skills and attitudes of a competent teacher.

Relationships with patients

- The doctor–patient partnership
- Good communication
- Children and young people
- Relatives, carers and partners
- Being open and honest with patients if things go wrong
- Maintaining trust in the profession
- Consent
- Confidentiality
- Ending your professional relationship with a patient.

This section covers the following areas in detail: listening to patients, sharing information, effective communication, awareness of the needs and welfare of children and young people, safeguarding and protecting the health and wellbeing of children and young people, being honest and open with patients when things go wrong, and consent and confidentiality.

Working with colleagues

- Working in teams
- Conduct and performance of colleagues
- Respect for colleagues
- Arranging cover
- Taking up and ending appointments
- Delegation and referral.

Working in teams does not change your personal accountability for your professional conduct and the care you provide. The need to act as a positive role model is emphasized in this section, as is the need to protect patients from harm posed by another colleague's conduct, performance or health. Suitable cover arrangements when off duty and effective handover procedures are essential. When delegating care or treatment you must be satisfied that the person to whom you delegate has the necessary qualifications, experience and skills to provide the care or treatment involved.

Probity

- Being honest and trustworthy
- Providing and publishing information about your services
- Writing reports and CVs, giving evidence and signing documents
- Research
- Financial and commercial dealings
- Conflicts of interest.

Being honest, trustworthy and acting with integrity are at the heart of medical professionalism. This should apply to published information about you and your services, in reports and documents you write or sign, in evidence that you give as a witness, with respect to any restrictions in your practice or suspensions anywhere in the world.

If you are involved in designing, organizing or carrying out research, you must put the protection of the participants' interests first, act with honesty and integrity and follow the appropriate national research governance guidelines.

You must be honest and open in any financial arrangements with patients and in financial and commercial dealings with employers, insurers and other organizations. You must act in your patients' best interests when making referrals and when providing or arranging treatment.

Health

The guidance is clear. You should be registered with a general practitioner outside your family to ensure that you have access to independent and objective medical care. You should not treat yourself. You should protect your patients, your colleagues and yourself by being immunized against common serious communicable diseases where vaccines are available.

If you know that you have, or think that you might have, a serious condition that you could pass on to patients, or if your judgement or performance could be affected by a condition or its treatment, you must consult a suitably qualified colleague. You must ask for and follow their advice about investigations, treatment and changes to your practice that they consider necessary. You must not rely on your own assessment of the risk you pose to patients.

Further reading

GMC. (2006). *Good Medical Practice*: http://www.gmc-uk.org (accessed 12 October 2010).

GMC supplementary guidance: http://www.gmc-uk.org (accessed 12 October 2010).

- Confidentiality 2009
- Consent 2008
- Conflicts of interest 2008
- Raising concerns about patient safety 2006
- Good practice in prescribing medicines 2006
- Good practice in decision making 2002
- Research: the role and responsibilities of doctors 2002

Guidelines

A guideline is a set of recommendations, based on best available evidence, that are designed to improve the delivery of healthcare. They can relate to patient care on an individual basis or to populations of patients. Guidelines are intended to provide guidance to healthcare professionals but not to replace clinical judgement; they differ from protocols in that they do not suggest a mandatory pathway of care.

Potential benefits of guidelines

The potential benefits of guidelines include:

- Promotion of interventions or treatments of proven benefits leading to reduced morbidity and mortality, and improved quality of life. At the same time clinicians are alerted to interventions/treatments not supported by good evidence
- Greater consistency of care locally and nationally, benefiting patients. This is also associated with more efficient use of resources and optimization of value or money in delivery of healthcare
- Improved communication between patient and healthcare professionals, e.g. it is increasingly common for guidelines to be accompanied by a lay version for patients and the public. These empower patients and help them to make informed decisions
- Their usefulness in developing quality improvement activities and standards to assess the clinical practice of individual health professionals (acting as a reference point for audit of an individual's or hospital's practice)
- Positive impact on the development of national health policy by drawing attention to a wide variety of neglected patient groups, health problems or clinical services
- Supporting education of new staff and staff returning to practice
- Strengthening the multidisciplinary team.

Potential limitations of guidelines

The potential limitations of using guidelines include:

- Reduced clinical autonomy and overreliance on the guideline by healthcare professionals
- Incorrect guidance leading to potential harm to patients from inferior, ineffective or harmful practices. Incorrect guidance also has serious deleterious implications for healthcare professionals by allowing their practice to be assessed against an incorrect benchmark
- Clinical guidelines can have an adverse effect on public policy.

Inaccurate/ineffective guidelines can arise for a number of reasons:
- Lack of accurate scientific data on the subject
- Recommendations that are too strongly influenced by the personal experience or knowledge of those involved in developing the guideline
- Differing priorities of those involved in developing the guideline, e.g. balancing costs against the needs of patients.

Development of a clinical guideline

Guidelines are increasingly developed according to a standardized model involving several key steps:
- Identifying the need for a clinical guideline
- Identifying the healthcare professional who will use the guideline
- Convening and running a guideline development group
- Searching for evidence of clinical effectiveness for a treatment (using systematic reviews)
- Assessing the evidence about the clinical question or condition
- Translating the evidence into a recommendation
- External review of the guideline
- Amending the guideline following a consultation process
- Implementing the guideline.

It is also mandatory that a timetable is set for regular review of the guideline.

Useful sources of guidelines

There are many sources of guidelines available, most of which are accessible via the Internet. The main organizations in the UK involved in writing and publishing guidelines include:
- NICE – National Institute for Health and Clinical Excellence
- SIGN – Scottish Intercollegiate Guidelines Network
- GAIN – Guidelines and Audit Implementation Network
- CKS – Clinical Knowledge Summaries (formerly Prodigy)
- Professional organizations and Royal Colleges.

The National Library of Guidelines is a collection of guidelines for the NHS (http://www.library.nhs.uk/guidelinesfinder/, accessed 14 December 2010). It is based on the guidelines produced by NICE and other national agencies. The main focus of the Library is on guidelines produced in the UK, but where no UK guideline is available, guidelines from other countries are included in the collection.

Implementing guidelines

Once a guideline has been developed, the next and perhaps most formidable part of the process is implementation of the guideline into clinical practice. Hospitals and other organizations need effective strategies to facilitate the uptake of guidelines into clinical practice.

Various factors can affect how successfully a guideline is implemented. These include:

- Resistance to change by the medical team
- Lack of awareness of the guideline
- Quality of the guideline
- Characteristics of the healthcare setting, e.g. primary care or hospital
- Inadequate resources to prevent uptake of the guideline.

There is no single way to implement a guideline effectively. Specific strategies to implement a clinical guideline may be divided into two types: primary strategies involving mailing or publication of the actual guidelines, and secondary interventional strategies to reinforce the guidelines. These strategies are variably effective, with secondary strategies probably having the most impact. A multifaceted approach will probably lead to the greatest success, with appropriate consideration being given to available resources.

Appraisal of guidelines

Once in use in clinical practice, the effectiveness of a guideline must be assessed by meticulous audit. In addition, the guideline must be reviewed on a regular basis in light of new evidence.

Preparation of a curriculum vitae

A curriculum vitae (CV) is the conventional way to present information about an individual in a variety of contexts but most obviously when applying for a job. It should be a summary of education, skills, achievements and experience. Most NHS jobs now use the generic web-based application form, but for a variety of reasons it is still essential to have an up-to-date CV. These include:

- Maintaining a CV is an excellent way to keep track of all aspects of training/career progression and will make it easier to fill in the generic NHS application form
- Even if the generic NHS application form is used initially, some hospitals may ask for a copy of your CV before shortlisting/interview
- A CV is essential for future appraisal and revalidation
- A CV is essential if applying for jobs outside of the NHS, e.g. overseas or to work in private hospitals.

General points

Aside from presenting information about an individual, a CV is a response to a specific advert, therefore it is essential that a CV contains a degree of flexibility; different aspects can be emphasized in response to different adverts. Before each and every job application a CV should be reviewed thoroughly.

There are no hard and fast rules with regard to the presentation of a CV, but it may be useful to consider the following points:

- Endeavour to make a CV as concise as possible. There is no limit to the length of a CV, but the trend is increasingly towards shorter CVs. Be careful not to lose your real strengths and achievements in pages of irrelevant information
- Folders/binders/covers are probably unnecessary. Ensure the pages of your CV are attached together securely – do not use paperclips. It can be useful to include a 'footer' at the bottom of each page with your name in small font. This will help should the CV pages come apart
- Be consistent with prose, fonts and headings. Use a font that is recognizable and easy to read, usually size 10–12
- Be meticulous about spelling. Spell checkers will not always pick up errors (e.g. to/too/two; they're, their, there), so be meticulous about reading your CV to pick up errors.

Layout

There are many possible layouts – a suggested format is demonstrated below.

Personal details

In this section it is important to include all the relevant information that a human resources department would need to contact you.

- Name
- Address
- Email address
- Contact telephone numbers.

In this section it is also conventional to include details of GMC registration, national training number and defence union number.

Personal information such as date of birth, gender and marital status is not required and it is a matter of choice as to whether it is included in this section.

Undergraduate and postgraduate education/qualifications/prizes

- Include details of secondary school education and university attended
- Include details of all degrees/other qualifications, e.g. diplomas.

Be careful about including details such as ATLS (advanced trauma life support) courses – not everyone perceives these as qualifications.

Current position

In this section state your current role, including the date commenced. It is also useful to include an outline of roles and responsibilities in this post.

NB: It is useful to contain all of the above three sections on one initial page.

Career history

This section should be a chronological account of your career history. It is essential that any gaps are explained, e.g. maternity leave.

Experience and achievements

Rather than describing in detail every training module you have completed, it may be useful to divide this section into 'relevant' and 'additional' experience. You should aim to highlight the particular skills you have acquired that are relevant to the job application in question.

Details of courses such as ATLS, etc. should be included here. This section should not be exhaustive and probably should be no longer than one to two sides of A4.

Audit

In the context of supporting clinical governance, audit is increasingly important. However, only include details of any audits where the audit loop has been closed.

Management/teaching experience

There is increasing emphasis on learning and developing management/leadership skills while still a trainee. There are many in-hospital programmes supported by regional deaneries and if you have completed any of these, details must be provided.

Equally if you have taken part in any formal teaching it should be included here.

Publications

This section should be subdivided if possible:

- Abstracts presented at scientific meetings (poster or verbal presentations)
- Abstracts published
- Original articles (including original research, case reports, editorials, continuing professional development (CPD) articles, etc.)
- Books/book chapters
- Published letters.

Outside interests

This is often a difficult part of a CV. The all-consuming nature of a medical career can sometimes leave little time to develop hobbies, but it is important that employers know that you can switch off!

If you take part in an activity/hobby outside of medicine that has benefits that can carry over into working life (e.g. playing sport in a team) or if you have an unusual hobby/interest, these can all be talking points in an interview.

Referees

Think carefully about who you will ask to be your referees and well in advance of any job application. Ensure that you ask whether they are happy to act as a referee for you and provide them with a copy of your CV. Make sure their contact details are accurate so that a human resources department is able to contact them easily.

A final appraisal of your CV

When your CV is finished it is worth doing two things. Firstly, read through it carefully and make sure that it gives the right impression and demonstrates clearly your ability to do the job. Secondly, it is always worth asking an independent person to make suggestions/constructive criticisms.

The final point to make is that it is good practice always to accompany your CV with a brief covering letter. The covering letter should succinctly introduce you and state the main reasons for your application and suitability for the post.

Chapter 10

Medical interviews

There are several hurdles to a successful medical career: these include success at a training programme interview for junior doctors, passing postgraduate examinations and success at the consultant interview.

Want the job

If you feel that you have trained for the post for which you are applying, you will perform much better than those who apply for a job about which they are ambivalent. Interviews are competitive and it is very rare for the best qualified candidate not to interview well and be offered the job. Therefore, your experience and relevant skills should be visible and clearly outlined in your curriculum vitae (CV). A post with a specialist interest should have an application form that mirrors the requirements of the post.

Job description

The post, its duties and responsibilities, will be available with the application form. The job plan will also be included and, if the candidate feels that he or she may offer some extra skills or wish for some minor amendments to the post, it is best to discuss these with the relevant clinical director or specialty lead prior to applying for the post. Interviews become awkward for the panel and the interviewee if these discussions are left to the time of the interview.

The internal candidate issue

Many jobs have an internal candidate, and prospective external candidates are put off a post for which they are well skilled by the mutterings of an 'idle grapevine' which will suggest that they have no chance because they are competing against a candidate for whom the post has been created. This type of rumour should be ignored. It is, generally, untrue and occasionally the job 'certainty' is not even shortlisted. All those who attend interviews are well aware that the favoured 'local candidate' who does not perform his or her best on the day will not be appointed. The candidate who performs best is invariably appointed and the committee is structured to ensure that this happens. Occasionally two excellent candidates appear for one job and both interview well. It is not uncommon for the local hospital to make a decision to create a second post on the day and, with the approval of the relevant Royal College representative, to appoint two worthy and chosen candidates. A candidate will always regret not applying for a job that he or she wants.

Dress and behaviour

Dress well. Behave professionally with everyone you meet.

Pre-interview visits

It is in your interests to understand the post and meet the relevant members of the trust for whom you hope to work. You must meet the relevant clinical director, any specialty lead and your future colleagues to familiarize yourself with the post. Are you suitable? What can you offer them? Where do you see the post developing over the next 5 or so years? Occasionally, a candidate visits his or her potential colleagues but is bereft of questions to ask them. This is your chance to understand what they wish from you. They also want to know about you, so take your CV along so they can see how suitable you are for the post.

A candidate must request a visit to the medical director and the trust chief executive if the interview is for a consultant post. This is the main chance for a candidate to find out what the major issues are in the trust. These can be financial, staffing, foundation trust status matters, or departmental in nature. It is important for the candidate to stress how willing he or she is to assist in the management of the trust as well as being enthusiastic about the specific post.

Know your curriculum vitae

Oddly enough candidates at interview seem to struggle to remember their CVs and therefore it is worth accentuating that this is the primary basis of the application and it should be known backwards.

The panel

The panel, especially for consultant posts, consists of a mixture of clinicians and management staff. There is a trust lay person who normally chairs the committee. A member of the human resources team within the hospital takes notes for future reference during the interviews in case there is an appeal by a candidate about any issues or questions raised in the interview. A Royal College assessor whose job is to ensure that all candidates are suitably qualified for the post is present. He or she provides information about the interview back to the relevant College. The clinicians are normally local doctors and future departmental colleagues. The medical director and chief executive or their delegates attend. Panels comprise about seven or eight interviewers for most interviews.

The interview

Interviews take about 45 minutes to conduct, with each interviewer asking the same two or three questions to each candidate. The Royal College representative asks about the candidate's CV with special relevance to the job, and the candidate must be able to present his or her career succinctly, accentuating relevant skills and talents. The local clinicians often ask about relevant internal departmental issues. Trust issues and national NHS issues are discussed by the managerial interviewers and the chairperson often asks a question assessing the candidate's all-round skills. Private practice matters should never be discussed in an NHS interview. A knowledgeable candidate should have no questions to ask the panel at the end as all job discussions should have taken place prior to the interview.

A presentation

Some posts start with a candidate presentation on a relevant trust issue. Stay within the delegated timeframe. PowerPoint presentations should be succinct and relevant. There are normally questions to the candidate at the end of the presentation.

Successful or unsuccessful

The successful candidate can rejoice, but those who are unsuccessful should and can obtain feedback about their performance from a local member of the panel. This is often most helpful to the candidate.

Core knowledge

Role of the consultant

Both the British Medical Association (BMA) and the Hospital Consultants and Specialists Association have defined the role of the medically qualified consultant in the modern NHS for the following reasons:

- A defined role would serve to indicate who should become consultants
- The role would shape the grounds on which consultants' performance is judged
- An understanding of the role is important when systems of care are being developed
- The role is intertwined in current debates on a post-CCT sub-consultant grade.

The role of the doctor theme was brought into focus by Professor Sir John Tooke in his report 'Aspiring to Excellence' in 2008. Recommendation 5 of the Tooke report states that:

> There needs to be a common shared understanding of the roles of all doctors in the contemporary healthcare team that takes due account of public expectations . . . Clarity of the doctor's role must extend to service contribution of the doctor in training, doctors currently contributing as locums, staff grades and associate specialists, the CCT-holder, the GP and the consultant.

Consultants are often singled out by a mixture of abilities: clinical skills involve taking on the most complex cases; management aspects involve the development of a service and the leadership of it; training provision requires the dissemination of professional knowledge and expertise to others. The BMA has defined a consultant as one who does the following:

- Provides high level specialist clinical input for patients in their care, including carrying out complex procedures and managing complex cases. A consultant is expected to be able to practise independently and autonomously, with competence in managing the vast majority of scenarios that could occur in their specialty
- Bears ultimate responsibility for patients under their care, including where care is delivered as part of a patient's pathway through multidisciplinary care
- Offers a specialist opinion for other teams on an area of subspecialization or personal academic interest
- Acts as an influential patient advocate within the healthcare system
- Provides leadership to multiple team areas of trust activity
- Quality assures their practice and that of the teams they lead, through clinical audit, appraisal and revalidation
- Provides, leads and oversees training and education for junior doctors, medical students and perhaps other healthcare professionals at both local and national levels
- Devises, reviews and revises organizations' policies, objectives, rules, working practices and protocols

- Conducts medical research in the public sector and/or private sector
- Promotes new practices and leads innovation in new models of care for patients, new forms of treatments and use of new technologies
- Practises medical management.

When defining the role of the consultant, it is clear that one size does not fit all. Different specialties have different attributes and the specific activities undertaken by consultants will vary depending on the individual's job plan. It is also impossible for consultants to practise everything in the role description to the same level all the time. The concept of 'stages to the consultant career' was first recognized in the NHS White Paper (2000) and lately by the Hospital Consultants and Specialists Association in their paper 'The Future Role of the NHS Consultant'. The suggestion in both papers is that consultants carry a greater part of the clinical workload in the early years and, with increasing seniority, emphasis be placed on teaching, research, management, working for professional bodies and wider NHS roles.

Clinical excellence and expertise

Clinical expertise is the primary attribute of a medical consultant. The primary objective of a consultant is to use expert knowledge and skill to diagnose and treat patients while retaining ultimate clinical responsibility for their care. As medical professionals, consultants have a responsibility for the expansion of their knowledge base, for its proper application and for its transmission to future practitioners. Consultants must have an ongoing commitment to the continuous improvement of their practice through continuous professional development. They must be able to demonstrate a commitment to inquire into and review the clinical outcomes of their work and to have those audits scrutinized by their peers. Delivery of the best healthcare does not only depend on accurate diagnosis and treatment – effective communication between the consultant and the patient is also essential. Consultants need to be able to communicate clearly with patients to allow them to make informed choices about their treatment. Consultants also act as the patient's advocate. Advocacy includes the provision of guidance and support through complex care pathways.

Managerial skills and leadership

Consultants are the key players in NHS clinical teams and are needed to manage and lead the service. They play an important role in setting priorities, developing policies and making other management decisions within their own departments and hospitals. By virtue of their longevity in post and their understanding of the day-to-day core business, both as leaders of individual services and in the wider context of hospital management, consultants are key to continuity in hospitals. Consultants must be able to work in partnership with the wider healthcare team and also in partnership with other consultants. At a higher organizational level, increasingly emphasis is placed on engagement of doctors in the management and leadership of health services. The chief executive of the NHS has called for the shortlist for every trust chief executive post to have a clinician on it within 3–5 years.

Leading change and innovation

As well as leadership of services and healthcare professionals, consultants provide leadership and innovation to pioneer and drive forward new treatments and models of care for patients. In December 2001, the BMA published the report 'Pioneers in Patient Care:

Consultants Leading Change'. This report highlighted the key role played by consultants in pioneering improvements in patient care. The NHS needs consultants as innovators of change to drive medicine forward.

Training the next generation

Consultants play an indispensable role as educators and possess the range of skills that doctors in training need to acquire. The role that consultants play in teaching and training has been identified by the GMC as a key attribute in its guidance *The Doctor as Teacher*. Consultants are also involved in the planning and quality assurance of training at a national level through their work with the Royal Colleges, GMC/PMETB (the Postgraduate Medical Education and Training Board) and other bodies promoting quality and professional standards in postgraduate medical education.

Further reading

British Medical Association Central Consultants and Specialists Committee. (2008). *The Role of the Consultant* www.bma.org.uk/careers/ becoming_doctor/roleofconsultant0708.jsp (accessed 8 May 2010).

Hospital Consultants and Specialists Association. (2008). *What's in a Name? The Future Role of the NHS Consultant – An HCSA Position Paper*. www.hcsa.com (accessed 8 May 2010).

Chapter °

Chairing meetings

Every meeting needs a chairperson to direct the proceedings. The chairperson has the authority to regulate the meeting and is responsible for enforcing any rules that govern the proceedings and the successful completion of business. A number of different rules, such as company rules and statutory regulations, govern the selection of a chairperson for a formal meeting.

Characteristics of a good chairperson

A good chairperson requires diplomacy and leadership skills, knowledge and experience, impartiality and objectiveness, and an ability to delegate and make decisions.

Responsibility of chairperson

The chairperson is responsible for making sure that each meeting is planned effectively, conducted according to the constitution and that matters are dealt with in an orderly and efficient manner. Before accepting the position, the chairperson must make sure that he/she will be available for all meetings – apologies for absence should not usually include the chairperson! The chairperson's role before, during and after a meeting is outlined below.

Before the meeting

- Plan the agenda. Include items brought by other members
- Identify which agenda items are for information, discussion or decision
- Be well briefed about each item and actions taken since the last meeting

Table 12.1 Characteristics of a good chairperson

A good chairperson will	A good chairperson will not
Make all members feel valued	Be the person who talks most at the meetings
Strive for consensus	Make all the decisions
Listen to others	Allow one or two people to dominate
Make new members feel welcome	Make people feel foolish or useless
Keep calm	Lose his/her temper
Keep control and focus	Allow meetings to become unproductive

- Ensure all necessary background papers and last meeting's minutes are sent out with the agenda
- Check that all practical arrangements have been made, e.g. room layout, visual aids
- Arrive in good time for the meeting.

During the meeting

- Communicate
    - Start the meeting. Welcome any new members. Make any necessary introductions
    - Receive apologies for absence
    - Ensure that additions or amendments to minutes are recorded
    - Set the scene. State the objectives of the meeting
    - Try to be brief when communicating a point
- Control
    - Set out time limits
    - Ensure quorum is present
    - Keep to the agenda
    - Allow flexibility and freedom of expression
    - Ensure time is used effectively
    - Ensure that minutes are taken
- Coax
    - Ensure full participation
    - Draw out quieter members and discourage those who are monopolizing the meeting
    - Be prepared to highlight issues and ask awkward questions
- Compare
    - Weigh up contributions impartially
    - All points in favour of a point should be summarized against all points not in favour
- Clarify
    - Ensure everyone understands what is being discussed
    - Summarize
    - Ensure that action plans are recorded, together with who is going to implement them
- Guide
    - Steer members to work harmoniously and purposefully as a team
    - Keep an eye on time
- Make decisions
    - Ensure that decisions are taken in the context of the organization's strategy and that they are recorded, together with who is going to implement them
    - Ensure that decisions are based on relevant information and an understanding of available choices and constraints.

At the end of the meeting

- Summarize decisions taken and action points to be followed by whom and by when
- Agree a date for the next meeting. It may be best to set dates for the year's meetings well in advance

- Agree on future business
- Set next agenda
- Ensure that minutes are written up, checked and sent out in good time.

Managing how committee members work together

The goal is to develop some guidelines or structures that facilitate the work of the committee. As early as possible, committee members should discuss the policies and procedures that the committee will use, such as when meetings will be held, how often they should be, what ground rules the committee will follow and how the committee will come to a decision. The decision procedure can vary depending on the issue and on the importance of the decision. Committees often come to a decision through majority vote, unanimous decision, weighted decision, multi-voting or criteria-based voting.

Dealing with disruptive behaviour

Problems of order at a meeting may arise from breaches of procedure, conflicts of interest or even wilful disruption. Examples include talking out of turn, side conversing, provoking argument, adopting negative and hostile attitudes, being abusive, unruly or violent. The chairperson must ensure that the meeting is conducted in an orderly fashion and restore calm if tempers become frayed. The nature of a meeting determines the limits or extent of the powers of a chairperson and the types of procedure that can be used to maintain order. The latter can range from addressing individuals directly and guiding the discussion back to the issues and away from those involved, to requesting trouble-makers to leave, to ejecting trouble-makers, to using legal procedures.

Dealing with poor attendance

Many committees have problems with poor attendance. This makes it difficult for committees to apply consistent, good quality, collective decision-making. Where committees are anxious not to lose valued members, many struggle to deal with this issue and are reluctant to take the necessary steps to improve attendance. The chairperson is responsible for dealing with poor attendance. He/she must find out what the constitution says about attendance and apply the rules.

Here are some common reasons for poor attendance:

- An issue in the member's work or personal life is temporarily absorbing much of their time and energy
- The member is busy and meeting attendance is never a priority
- The member is finding it difficult to participate effectively
- Meetings are not purposeful or productive so the member does not see much point in attending
- Meetings are so unfriendly that the member does not want to be part of it.

Some suggested approaches to poor attendance include:

- Developing a code of conduct for members
- Providing committee members with role descriptions, specifying the required commitment
- Reviewing who is on the committee and recruitment strategies

- Reviewing length of tenure
- Reviewing how meetings are run, their frequency, how decisions are made, use of alternative means of communication, etc.
- Using team-building activities to build relationships and commitment
- Ensuring shared focus around roles in relation to the organization's vision, mission and values.

Chapter 13

Educational supervision

The educational supervisor role has come to prominence following the implementation of 'Modernising Medical Careers', which introduced shorter, more focused, competency-based postgraduate training programmes. The importance of the role of educational supervisor is emphasized in the GMC publication *The New Doctor*, produced in conjunction with the Postgraduate Medical Education and Training Board (PMETB) and the *Gold Guide* to postgraduate specialty training in the UK. The role is now well defined and no longer considered a mere 'add on' for busy consultants and general practitioners. It is a role that has to be planned, protected and valued. Increasingly, educational supervisors will be professionally selected, trained and paid for their work. They will also be held to account for standards of practice as defined by the PMETB, as education and training become ever more quality assured.

Role definitions

Clinical supervision relates to day-to-day oversight of trainees in the workplace and is an activity that involves all clinicians that come into contact with trainees. Clinical supervision involves being available, looking over the shoulder of the trainee, teaching on-the-job with developmental conversations, regular feedback and the provision of a rapid response to issues as they arise. All trainees should have access to supervision at all times with the degree of supervision tailored to their competence, confidence and experience. Within a given training placement, and for each trainee, such arrangements may be the responsibility of a nominated clinical supervisor.

The PMETB defines a clinical supervisor as a 'trainer who is selected and appropriately trained to be responsible for overseeing a specified trainee's clinical work and providing constructive feedback during a training placement'.

Educational supervision relates to the oversight of a trainee's progress over time. Educational supervisors are responsible for ensuring that trainees are making the necessary clinical and educational progress. They need all the skills of clinical supervision, plus an appreciation of supporting educational theory, an ability to undertake appraisal, work with portfolios, provide careers advice and manage the trainee in difficulty with support from deanery training structures.

The PMETB defines an educational supervisor as a 'trainer who is selected and appropriately trained to be responsible for the overall supervision and management of a specified trainee's educational progress during a training placement or series of placements. The Educational Supervisor is responsible for the trainee's Educational Agreement'.

Role and responsibilities

According to the *Gold Guide*, educational supervisors should:

- Be adequately prepared for the role and have an understanding of educational theory and practical educational techniques
- Be trained to offer educational supervision and undertake appraisal and feedback
- Undertake training in competence assessment for specialty training
- Be trained in equality and diversity
- Provide regular appraisal opportunities, which should take place at the beginning, middle and end of a placement
- Develop a learning agreement and educational objectives with the trainee, which is mutually agreed and is the point of reference for future appraisal
- Ensure that trainees whom they supervise maintain and develop their specialty learning portfolio and participate in the specialty assessment process
- Provide regular feedback to the trainee on their progress
- Ensure that the structured report, which is a detailed review and synopsis of the trainee's learning portfolio, is returned within the necessary timescales
- Contact the employer (usually the medical director) and the Postgraduate Dean in case the level of performance of a trainee is of concern
- Advise the trainee about access to career management
- Be responsible for their educational role to the Training Programme Director and locally to the employer's lead for postgraduate medical education.

Dealing with the challenging trainee

The challenging trainee is one who takes up a disproportionate amount of the educational supervisor's time. This includes trainees with attitude problems, communication difficulties, unrealistic expectations, bullying tendencies and extends to trainees with serious psychiatric disorders. An extremely important role for the educational supervisor is to be part of the mechanism for identifying problems early and being able to put in place the support mechanisms to prevent any further deterioration. Challenging trainees can be identified in many ways. Some of the most common signs are a change in attitude at work, deteriorating clinical performance, isolation from peer group, increasing time off sick or turning up late for work. If the educational supervisor is made aware of any performance outside the acceptable limits of practice, they must arrange a prompt meeting with the trainee. After the reflective discussion, there needs to be a specific agreed plan and an assessment of progress. An ongoing log of accurate documentation is essential. It is very important that educational supervisors know where to seek advice and to whom a trainee should be referred in the case of serious performance, conduct and patient safety issues.

Selection and accreditation of supervisors

The London Deanery requires all educational supervisors to be selected for their role, participate in the 3-yearly educational review process and demonstrate that they have undertaken training in the appropriate areas of the Deanery Professional Development Framework. In addition, the London Deanery expects that all supervisors should refresh their training in equal opportunities and diversity every 3 years and those involved in the recruitment process should attend interview and/or selection skills training.

The Deanery expects all trusts to implement mandatory training and a developmental system of 3-yearly appraisal and review of all educational supervisors. The review must include a formal statement of accreditation from the Director of Medical Education (or nominated deputy). Trust and other local education providers must provide an ongoing programme of faculty development in accordance with the identified development needs of all educators within the trust or provider.

Local faculty development programmes

Rolling programmes of faculty development must be provided within each trust to enable clinical or educational supervisors to meet mandatory training requirements. Supervisors who wish to pursue their educational development in more depth can enrol on a university accredited course such as the MA in Clinical Education at the Institute of Education (www. ioe.ac.uk, accessed 8 November 2010) or on courses that are offered by the Academy of Medical Educators (www.medicaleducators.org, accessed 8 November 2010). In future years, it is envisaged that the professional standards for 'faculty' will continue to rise to the level that exists in general practice, where potential trainers undertake a modular postgraduate teaching programme before applying to train.

Educational tariff

From 2010, the PMETB requires that trainers have a suitable job plan with an appropriate workload and time to develop trainees. It is therefore now an expectation in educational contracts with trusts that appropriate time for training is allocated within an individual consultant's job plan. This is monitored as part of a Deanery's routine quality and contract monitoring processes.

Educational supervisor portfolio documentation

It is now mandatory for educational supervisors to maintain a portfolio demonstrating a professional, informed and coherent approach to the supervision of trainees. The following information should be presented within the portfolio:

- Personal information
- Description of the role
- Prior accreditation or experience (conditional grandfather clause, if applicable)
- Training courses relevant to supervisory role
- Evidence of good practice
- Personal development plan.

Summary

Every doctor in training should have an educational supervisor. Educational supervision can be demanding, time-consuming and sometimes a stressful responsibility. However, it is very often a positive experience for the trainee and the supervisor and, in the longer term, a successful educational supervisor network raises the profile of a hospital and assists recruitment at all levels.

Further reading

A Guide to Postgraduate Specialty Training in the UK – The Gold Guide (2007). www.mmc.nhs.uk (accessed 24 April 2010).

Cooper, N. and Forrest, K. (2009). *Essential Guide to Educational Supervision in Postgraduate Medical Education*. UK: Wiley–Blackwell.

Department of Health. (2008). *A High Quality Workforce. NHS Next Stage Review*. London: Department of Health.

Professional Development Framework for Supervisors in the London Deanery (2009). www.londondeanery.ac.uk (accessed 24 April 2010).

Core skills

Effective delegation

Delegation is an art – it builds trust, develops skills in those to whom tasks have been delegated and frees the delegator to work on other priorities. Effective delegation is fundamental to leadership and time management. In clinical practice, delegation involves asking a colleague to provide treatment or care on your behalf. Although you will not be accountable for the decisions and actions of those to whom you delegate, you are still responsible for the overall management of the patient and accountable for your decision to delegate.

Why delegate?

There are many obvious benefits to delegation:

- It shows you have faith in the people with whom you work
- It gives you more time to focus on important activities
- It utilizes your management skills
- It helps to develop and motivate staff
- It transfers work to individuals whose skills in a particular area are better than yours.

What stops you?

- Unwillingness or inability to 'let go' – owing either to a fear of surrendering authority or because you like to give the impression of being overworked
- Perfectionism – owing to a lack of confidence in another's abilities and your fear of mistakes
- Belief that others 'are not up to the job' – you fear that others will under-perform
- You enjoy 'getting your hands dirty' – you get satisfaction doing jobs yourself and you get them done effectively
- Lack of time – you feel that jobs may take longer to achieve with delegation and could be accomplished quicker if you did them yourself
- Guilt – you feel guilty for imposing more work on colleagues or junior members of staff
- Fear of becoming unpopular – you fear what others may think of you
- Your ego.

How to delegate

There are clear steps to delegation and if you delegate with honourable intentions people will not think the worse of you.

Decide what to delegate

One way of deciding what to delegate is simply to list the things you do which could be more effectively done by someone who is either more skilled in a particular area or less expensive. Alternatively, you may wish to use your activity log, which will show you where you are spending large amounts of time on low yield jobs. You should consider delegating things you are good at, things you are bad at and work which will provide experience. You should not be delegating ultimate responsibility for the task nor should you use delegating as a means of ridding yourself of all the jobs you dislike.

Select capable and willing people

How far you can delegate jobs will depend on the ability, experience and reliability of individuals. Choose a person who would really enjoy the task and who has the appropriate skills or willingness to learn them. Also select those that you can trust and make them feel an important part of the process. When you delegate care or treatment you must be satisfied that the person to whom you delegate has the qualifications, experience, knowledge and skills to provide the care or treatment necessary.

Provide context

It is essential to be clear about what is required and why it is important. Let them see and understand the bigger picture. Explain how the work you are delegating contributes to the overall success of the team. Framing the delegated work within the broader context energizes recipients.

Brief

Ensure that you communicate effectively the results that are needed, the constraints within which it should be carried out, the deadlines for completion and internal reporting dates when you want information on the progress of the task or project. When delegating in clinical practice, always pass on enough information about the patient and the treatment they need. The process of delegating is not complete until the recipient of the information feels confident and able to undertake the work alone.

Delegate authority

This can be difficult for many as it requires confidence in the individual. Yet without the necessary authority for decision-making, people will not be empowered to complete the tasks they have been given. If appropriate, make other people aware that you have delegated authority to your colleague.

Support – don't abdicate

Delegation does not mean complete withdrawal. Particularly in the early stages, people need support and encouragement to take on additional responsibility. Abdication can leave the delegated person feeling isolated.

Monitor progress

Checking progress and providing constructive feedback are crucial. How much you monitor will depend upon the capability and experience of the person to whom you have delegated.

Evaluate results

This is a time of reflection on your part. Consider whether you delegated successfully.

Give credit when a job has been successfully completed

Although this may seem obvious it can be forgotten. Always acknowledge a person's contribution on completion of the task.

Summary

Effective delegation allows you to make the best use of your time and it helps other people in the team to grow and develop to reach their full potential in the organization. Probably the most important reason for delegating is to develop the skills of other people as well as your own. Senior doctors have a responsibility to develop everyone in the team and all junior doctors deserve the opportunity to develop their skills. Delegation is a vital skill for team leaders and, like any skill, it must be learned and practised. There are times when the project is too important to pass on to others and times when you are the best person for the job. To delegate effectively, choose the right tasks to delegate, identify the right people to delegate to, and delegate in the right way.

Further reading

Christie, S (2009). *Effective Time Management Skills for Doctors*, Nottingham: Developmedica.

GMC. (2006). *Good Medical Practice* London: GMC.

Chapter 15

Leadership styles

From Mahatma Gandhi to Winston Churchill to Martin Luther King, there are as many leadership styles as there are leaders. Fortunately, business people and psychologists have developed useful and simple ways to describe the main styles of leadership and these can help aspiring leaders to understand which styles they should adopt. So, whether you manage a team at work, captain a sports team or lead a major organization, which approach is best?

Autocratic leadership

With this form of leadership leaders have absolute power over their workers or team. At one extreme, these leaders are aloof from their staff, thinking big thoughts, their eye on the distant horizon, focused exclusively on their task and their destiny to remake the world in their own image. They will have total authority over any decision-making and tell their followers what needs to be done and how the tasks should be completed. Staff and team members have little opportunity to make suggestions. A variation of this type of leadership is known as 'command and compliance', a style that does have its place and its uses. It is particularly effective when time is limited, such as in a medical emergency when it is vital for someone to take charge and prevent any chaos or confusion. Another example is when a doctor prescribes a course of antibiotics for a medical condition and the patient is advised to take the medicine. The style is also good when dealing with groups that need close supervision, such as young children or very inexperienced employees and recruits.

Bureaucratic leadership

These leaders work 'by the book'. They follow rules rigorously and ensure that their staff follow procedures precisely. This is a very appropriate style for work involving serious safety risks or the handling of money. This type of leader is also able to make use of organizational systems to provide them with control and power. These leaders are to be found throughout the NHS.

Democratic leadership

This kind of style prioritizes team participation, with the leader allowing each member to contribute ideas. These leaders are focused on their people and their staff. They do not seek aggrandisement for themselves, just progress for their constituency. Their style is consensual and discursive. This type of participative leadership is evident in clinical decision-making within multidisciplinary teams. This style not only motivates and increases job satisfaction in teams, but also helps to develop people's skills. One drawback of this leadership style is that it can make it difficult to make quick decisions when time is short or there is an emergency.

Laissez-faire leadership

This French phrase means 'leave it be', and it is used to describe leaders who leave their team members to work on their own. With this leadership style followers are effectively given free rein to make decisions and do what they think is appropriate. Although this sounds risky, this leadership style can work if team members are highly experienced and require little supervision to achieve the expected outcome. To be effective, the leader needs to monitor what is being achieved and communicate this back to the team regularly.

Task-oriented leadership

Task-oriented leaders focus only on getting the job done. They actively define the work and the roles required, put structures in place, plan, organize and monitor. This approach can suffer many of the flaws of autocratic leadership, with difficulties in motivating and retaining staff.

People-oriented leadership

This is the opposite of task-oriented leadership. These leaders are totally focused on organizing, supporting and developing their teams. It is a participative style and tends to encourage good teamwork and creative collaboration.

Transactional leadership

This type of leader is focused on the business of the organization. Their goal is to maintain the status quo. They are seen as keeping an existing service running smoothly and providing stability to services in the face of change.

Transformational leadership

This style is creative, visionary and proactive. The status quo is no longer enough. These leaders have the talents required to manage change in the organization. In many organizations, both transactional and transformational leaders are needed. The transactional leaders ensure that routine work is done reliably, while the transformational leaders embrace initiatives that add new value.

Summary

There is no 'right' way to lead. Each style of leadership will have varying degrees of success in different situations. Effective leaders often switch instinctively between styles, according to the people they lead and the work that needs to be accomplished. Successful leadership is more often a question of finding the right approach for a particular situation or setting.

Chapter 16

Leadership competences

No single area of organizational behaviour has been more researched and debated than leadership and management. There are many who would argue that leadership and management are interchangeable terms. However, there are important differences between the two. In lay terms, leadership is about giving guidance by going in front; management is about conducting or controlling a business or enterprise.

In the NHS the two terms tend to be used in different ways. A leader is someone who has a vision about how hospitals, departments or teams should develop or change and is able to drive the change; leaders take people with them towards the objectives they have set and create an environment in which people can develop. Leadership is a key part of doctors' professional work regardless of specialty and setting. You do not have to be a consultant or a chief executive to exercise leadership. For example, anyone who has had to deal with a busy on-call or leads a ward round or initiates and implements change would be demonstrating leadership.

Management is a different process, with a different purpose.

Table 16.1 Leadership versus management

Leader	Manager
Concerned with doing the right thing	Concerned with doing things right
Takes the long-term view	Takes the short-term view
Thinks in terms of innovations, development and the future	Thinks in terms of administration, maintenance and the present
Sets the vision: the tone and direction	Sets the plan: the pace
Hopes others will respond and follow	Hopes others will complete their tasks
Expects others to help realize a vision	Expects others to fulfil their mission or purpose
Inspires innovation	Inspires stability

The importance of developing leadership competences as an integral part of a doctor's training and learning is now well recognized. It is already a requirement of all doctors, as laid out in the GMC publications *Good Medical Practice* and *Management for Doctors*. Professor Sir John Tooke, in his 2008 report 'Aspiring to Excellence', commented that 'The doctor's frequent role as head of the healthcare team and commander of considerable clinical resource requires that greater attention is paid to management and leadership skills regardless of specialism'.

The Medical Leadership Competency Framework (MLCF) has been developed as an aid and driver for the development of such skills. It has been jointly developed by the Academy of Medical Royal Colleges and the NHS Institute for Innovation and Improvement in conjunction with a wide range of stakeholders, and as part of the 'Enhancing Engagement in Medical Leadership' project. This UK-wide project aims to promote medical leadership and create organizational cultures where doctors seek to be more engaged in management and leadership of health services and non-medical leaders genuinely seek their involvement to improve services for patients across the UK. The framework describes the leadership competences doctors need to become more actively involved in the planning, delivery and transformation of health services. It is built on the concept of shared leadership, where leadership is not restricted to those who hold designated leadership roles. The MLCF applies to all medical students and doctors throughout their training and career. It is a pivotal tool which can be used to:

- Design training curricula and programmes
- Highlight an individual's strengths and development areas through both self-assessment and colleague feedback
- Help with personal development planning and career progression.

There are five domains in the MLCF. To deliver appropriate, safe and effective services, it is essential that any doctor is competent in each domain. Within each domain there are four elements and each of these elements is further divided into four competency outcomes.

Table 16.2 MLCF domains

Demonstrating personal qualities	Working with others
Developing self-awareness	Developing networks
Managing yourself	Building and maintaining relationships
Continuing personal development	Encouraging contribution
Acting with integrity	Working within teams
Managing services	**Improving services**
Planning	Ensuring patient safety
Managing resources	Critically evaluating
Managing people	Ensuring improvement and innovation
Managing performance	Facilitating transformation
Setting direction	
Identifying the contexts for change	
Applying knowledge and evidence	
Making decisions	
Evaluating impact	

Leadership opportunities for trainees

There are many resources and initiatives available to trainees who wish to develop leadership skills:

- Organizations and networks, e.g. Network With No Name, www.networkwithnoname. net (accessed 29 December 2010)
- Leadership development schemes, e.g. NHS London Prepare to Lead, www.london.nhs. uk/leading-for-health/programmes/prepare-to-lead (accessed 29 December 2010)
- Secondments and fellowships, e.g. NHS London Darzi Fellowships, Harkness Fellowships, secondments offered by McKinsey and Company, etc.
- Educational qualifications and courses, e.g. Masters in Medical Leadership, Warwick University; MBA at Keele University, etc.

Being a team leader

Team leadership is an important 'life skill' and role that needs to be understood, learned and practised. The primary task of the team leader is to ensure that team goals are achieved. This requires the team leader to project the vision, seek talent, build on diversity and develop colleagues within the team. The following approach will lend itself to effective team leadership in a variety of situations:

- Assess the people you are working with or select appropriate individuals for the task in hand
- Set clear direction
- Make sure that team objectives are understood by everyone
- Check the available resources
- Agree action plans and achievable deadlines
- Foster team spirit and sustain enthusiasm
- Maintain communication links
- Analyse and correct failures swiftly
- Acknowledge, publicize and celebrate team successes
- Carry the responsibility of representing the team loyally, both inside and outside the organization.

Summary

Doctors must be at the forefront of NHS leadership. They have a responsibility to contribute to the effective running of the organization in which they work and to its future direction. After all, if the dust ever has a chance to settle between cycles of change, the doctors will still be there.

Further reading

http://www.institute.nhs.uk/medicalleadership (accessed 15 September 2010).

Belbin, R.M. (2010). *Team Roles at Work*. Oxford: Butterworth–Heinemann.

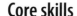

Mentoring

17

Mentoring is a very old concept in a new guise. It can be traced back to Greek mythology when Odysseus entrusted his son Telemachus to his old and trusted friend Mentor, who acted as a wise counsellor and helper to the youth. Mentoring then became common practice in the time of the guilds and trade apprenticeships when young people who had acquired technical skills often benefited from the patronage of more experienced and established professionals.

There are many opinions of what mentoring is or should be about. The traditional view is that it is based on a longlasting, usually spontaneous, relationship in which a more skilled or experienced person (the mentor) serves as a role model and supports, guides, advises, teaches, encourages, counsels and befriends a less skilled or experienced person in need of help for the purpose of promoting their professional and personal development. In recent years, newer models of mentoring have been developed where the emphasis is on mutual support rather than the flow of help in a single direction from mentor to mentee, and this is known as co-mentoring. One of the key ingredients in all mentoring arrangements is the skill of 'active listening'.

The definition of mentoring used most often in medicine comes from the Standing Committee on Postgraduate Medical and Dental Education: 'An experienced highly regarded empathic person (the mentor) guides another individual (the mentee) in the development and re-examination of his or her own ideas, learning, personal and professional developments. This is achieved by listening and talking in confidence.'

The aims of a mentoring relationship depend upon the needs of the mentee and can change over time as the mentee develops. Common examples of such needs include identifying career goals, developing action plans, exam and course guidance, research advice, help in preparing a CV and improving interview techniques.

Who needs mentoring?

Doctors at all stages of their careers can benefit from mentoring. However, those who need it most are those new to an organization or position, those concerned with aspects of their career, those being developed for future leadership positions, those in professional or personal difficulty and those with cultural barriers at work such as ethnic minority or overseas doctors. There is a perceived need for extra support for newly appointed GP principals, consultants, specialty doctors and foundation year trainees.

Benefits of mentoring
Benefits to the mentee

Mentees value the dedicated time for reflection during which someone they trust listens 'actively', challenges their thinking but does not problem-solve on their behalf. They also benefit by being supported and assisted in developing for themselves strategies for dealing with the specific issues that they raise with their mentors, by regaining self-confidence and feelings of self-worth, improved working relationships and job satisfaction.

Benefits to the mentor

Philosophically speaking, mentoring is a selfless act and no prospective mentor should indulge in it with self-benefit as the primary aim. Nevertheless, the process has some benefits for the mentor as well, which lie chiefly in the sharing of experiences and learning with junior colleagues and the sense of satisfaction that is derived from seeing the mentee develop. Some mentors find that the mentoring principles and skills set can be applied to many other areas of their practice.

Benefits to the organization

Mentoring helps doctors to feel valued and such doctors are more likely to provide better care to patients. It also provides an opportunity to identify doctors in difficulty at an early stage.

Qualities of a good mentoring relationship

The process of mentoring is essentially a relationship between two people and for it to succeed there must be a high level of mutual trust and respect between the two parties. The mentoring relationship should enable the mentee to learn and grow in a safe and protected environment. The quality of the relationship is crucial to a successful outcome. The boundaries on the relationship, in terms of its limits and duration, need to be defined and agreed. For good mentoring it is important that the approach of the mentor is constructive and non-judgemental and that the process is facilitative and developmental. Reflection should be an integral part of the mentoring process. Hay views the mentoring relationship as a 'life cycle' with four stages:

Stage 1: initiation, orientation or courtship – creating an alliance, bonding, setting objectives and defining an agenda.
Stage 2: honeymoon, getting established, adolescence, dependency and nurturing.
Stage 3: maturing, developing autonomy or independence.
Stage 4: ending, termination, divorce, closure.

A good mentor should have good interpersonal skills, adequate time, an open mind and a willingness to support the relationship. Medical mentors should also be knowledgeable about study leave guidelines, immigration and employment laws, grievance procedures and equal opportunities law. It is said that a mentor should Motivate, Empower and Encourage, Nurture self-confidence, Teach, Offer wise counsel and Raise the performance of the mentee.

Initiation of the mentoring relationship

In informal mentoring, the process is usually but not invariably initiated at the behest of the mentee. In structured mentoring the process often starts as part of an organizational policy or project. Only rarely does a mentoring relationship occur as a sole initiative of the mentor.

Mentorship schemes

For doctors wanting to become formal mentors with official recognition of this role in job plans, there are several mentorship programmes available through Deaneries, Royal

Colleges and other training and development organizations. Mentor networks and support events can provide ongoing mentor support. Organizations that do not provide their own mentoring arrangements should facilitate doctors' access to appropriate schemes.

How are mentors and mentees best matched?

Techniques for bringing mentors and mentees together formally vary considerably. They range from encouraging mentees to exercise free choice from a pool of potential mentors, all the way to allocation of the next available mentor from the top of a list. Some schemes are specialty-specific, with both mentor and mentee from the same discipline. Some employ personality measures (Myers–Briggs Type Indicator). Scheme organizers often exercise judgement about who will suit whom.

Difficulties with mentoring

Difficulties arise usually on account of improper conduct of the mentoring process. Improperly conducted mentoring can result in stress, role confusion and disillusionment with the task. A mentoring relationship may become dysfunctional as a result of personality traits that are not compatible with the process. In medicine, a junior doctor's mentor is often a consultant under whom the doctor works. This type of mentoring has been termed 'faculty mentoring'. This approach can often lead to a conflict of interest between the mentoring and supervisory roles of the mentor and consequently may interfere with the mentoring process.

Another potential downside of mentoring is that, over a period of time, mentors tend to acquire considerable personal and private knowledge about their mentees, which can lead to problems if confidentiality is not maintained. Safeguards for confidentiality are vital in maintaining the integrity of the mentoring process and should be observed at all times, barring exceptional circumstances when public safety may be at stake. Other difficulties that may be encountered during mentoring include frustration from lack of progress or conflicts.

Summary

Mentoring is an important developmental process and, carried out correctly, can enhance professional and personal life. There is a strong perception amongst both mentors and mentees that mentoring, if well conducted and well timed, can reap enormous benefits for the mentees and at the same time be useful to the mentors and the organization. The most commonly described benefit is personal – personal empowerment, personal functionality, personal growth. Mentoring is valuable for managing transition points in professional careers. Many government and medical organizations now support mentoring for doctors.

Further reading

Gupta, R.C. and Lingam, S. (2000). *Mentoring for Doctors and Dentists*. Oxford: Blackwell Science.

Hay, J. (1995). *Transformational Mentoring*. New York: McGraw-Hill.

Mentoring for doctors: signposts to current practice for career grade doctors (2004) www.dh.gov.uk/publications (accessed 7 May 2010).

Standing Committee on Postgraduate Medical and Dental Education (1998). *Supporting Doctors and Dentists at Work: An Enquiry into Mentoring*. London: SCOPME.

Taherian, K. and Shekarchian, M. (2008). Mentoring for doctors. Do its benefits outweigh its disadvantages? *Medical Teacher*, **30**(4): 95–9. Informa Healthcare.

18

Time management

How often do you find that you have too much to do and too little time in which to do it? As a doctor you face many pressures each day, with more and more people placing demands on your time. It seems that there is never enough time in the day to get everything done. There are many duties and responsibilities that require your time and attention and you may frequently feel yourself pulled in different directions. You have to organize your time around a long list of clinical duties such as ward rounds, clinics, operating theatre sessions, multidisciplinary team meetings and on-call work. You have administrative tasks such as writing up discharge summaries and reports, dictating clinic notes, responding to queries and complaints. The clinical environment today also requires you to undertake teaching, give presentations, attend meetings and cover for absent colleagues, while continuing with your own development as a doctor. For you to balance all these activities and enhance your personal effectiveness, self-organization is clearly required.

The term 'time management' is somewhat of a misnomer, as time itself cannot be managed. We can only manage ourselves and our use of time. Most doctors have the capacity to manage their time better and by doing so can make their working day more productive and leisure time more fulfilling. The introduction of the European Working Time Directive has made the need for effective time management critical for doctors in training.

Steps to effective time management

For you to manage your time better, you need to find out how it is currently being used and then consider how you can reallocate it in a more effective way. You can facilitate this by following these steps given below.

Assess your day

There are always competing demands on your time. It is very easy to spend too much time on routine things, such as reading emails, at the expense of high priority, productive tasks. Do you prioritize your work so that you tackle important and urgent projects first or do you concentrate on completing enjoyable tasks first?

Keep an activity log

Maintaining a time log of how much time you spend on particular activities is fundamental to managing your time more effectively. Keeping an activity log for several days or weeks will help you to understand how you spend your time.

Table 18.1 Prioritizing tasks

1	2
Urgent and important	**Important but not urgent**
'Fire-fighting'	'Quality time'
3	4
Urgent but not important	**Neither urgent nor important**
'Distraction'	'Time-wasting'

Analyse your activity log

This will enable you to identify and eliminate time-wasting or low yield jobs. Apply Pareto's principle to your activities. Vilfredo Pareto was an Italian economist who, in 1906, noted that 20% of the people owned 80% of the wealth in his country. Subsequently Joseph Juran, a quality management pioneer, recognized that 20% of something is always responsible for 80% of the results. Focus on the 20% of tasks that will bring you the greatest results.

Prepare 'to do' lists

This will remind you to carry out all necessary tasks. A 'to do' list should be a prioritized list with the important, urgent tasks at the top.

Prioritize tasks

Categorize them as indicated in Table 18.1. Consciously strive to maximize quadrant 2 time. Allocate time to carry out these tasks when you are at your best. Doing so can reduce the amount of time taken up by fire-fighting (quadrant 1) activities, since many quadrant 1 activities could have been quadrant 2 if they had been done earlier. You can also seek to reduce time spent in quadrant 3 by improving your systems and processes for dealing with distractions.

Identify time-stealers

These could be interruptions (telephone, visitors), unclear objectives, lack of planning and organization, tasks that could have been delegated, inadequate technical knowledge, unclear communications, incomplete information, poorly conducted and unproductive meetings, stress and fatigue, personal disorganization, office and desk clutter.

Be realistic

There are few things more stressful than exaggerated expectations, so be realistic about what you can achieve in a given period of time. Learn to recognize the limits of your capabilities and do not undertake a project that you know you cannot complete successfully.

Schedule quiet time

Time for yourself is necessary. Even a short period of relaxation will help you to work more efficiently. Keep some energy for home life and leisure activities after work. When energy is low, you are sluggish and will make mistakes.

Schedule refreshment breaks

Food and drink is vital for concentration levels.

Time tasks

It is important to allocate the most demanding tasks of the day to the times when you are at your best. Do not waste high energy time doing low priority work.

Handle interruptions

Ask yourself what is more important, the interruption or what you are working on? Try to keep interruptions short. Be assertive, learn to say 'no' and learn to deal with the 'have you got a minute' scenario.

Delegate aspects of your work

This is one of the keys to effective management as it allows you the time to complete the most important elements of your job.

Summary and key points

Time management is an essential skill that will help you to keep your work under control. As you follow the 12 steps and begin to organize your day into a meaningful structure your productivity will rise, stress levels will fall and you will regain confidence in your own abilities. Regaining control of your workload will create a very favourable impression of you as a competent doctor and earn you respect from those around you. You will also benefit personally as you regain a work–life balance that makes you a more rounded individual.

- Time management is about doing things more effectively, not more quickly
- Organize your time
- Time spent on drawing up a plan is never a waste – if you fail to plan, then plan to fail!
- Focus on goals
- Avoid distractions
- Organize your space
- Delegate effectively.

Further reading

Christie, S. (2009). *Effective Time Management Skills for Doctors*. Nottingham: Developmedica.

Hindle, T. (1998). *Manage Your Time*. London: Dorling Kindersley.

www.teal.org.uk (accessed 5 April 2010).

Chapter

19

General Medical Council

Role of the GMC

The General Medical Council (GMC) registers doctors to practise medicine in the UK. Its statutory purpose is to protect, promote and maintain the health and safety of the public by ensuring proper standards in the practice of medicine. The GMC has four distinct functions under the Medical Act 1983.

- Keeping up-to-date registers of qualified doctors – the register is made available to employers and the general public so the registration of doctors can be verified
- Fostering good medical practice – the GMC issues a range of guidance aimed at promoting high standards of care
- Promoting high standards of medical education – this is achieved by setting standards for medical schools and, together with the Postgraduate Medical Education and Training Board (PMETB), for postgraduate training programmes. The GMC also encourages doctors to keep up to date through continuous professional development
- Dealing firmly and fairly with doctors whose fitness to practise is in doubt.

The GMC was established under the Medical Act of 1858. It is a registered charity in England, Wales and Scotland. The governing body, the Council, has 24 members, of which 12 are doctors and 12 are lay members, all appointed by the Appointments Commission. As a UK-wide body, the GMC regulates doctors registered in all four countries of the UK and has devolved offices in Belfast, Edinburgh and Cardiff. The GMC also cooperates with a variety of other regulators and organizations representing patients and doctors. Niall Dickson, a former BBC journalist, editor of *Nursing Times* and chief executive of The King's Fund, joined the GMC as chief executive and registrar in January 2010.

Legislation

The functions of the GMC and the way it carries out its functions are set out in law. The most important piece of legislation is the Medical Act. This provides the legal basis for all its functions. Over time a range of legislation has been introduced that defines the GMC's powers and responsibilities. The GMC also has to comply with relevant European law. The arrangements for the governance of the GMC are also set out in legislation.

Registration and licence to practise

The Medical Act requires the GMC to keep the register of medical practitioners and gives it the powers to make regulations covering the content and maintenance of the register. The GMC therefore makes arrangements for granting registration and licences to practise, including the setting of the 'annual retention fee' payable by doctors for maintaining their name on the register. On 16 November 2009 the GMC introduced the licence to practise. To practise medicine in the UK all doctors are now required by law to hold both registration and a licence to practise. This applies whether they practise full time, part time, as a locum, privately or in the NHS. To retain their licence to practise, doctors will need to demonstrate to the GMC that they are up to date and fit to practise.

The Medical Act gives the GMC powers to erase a doctor's name from the register for various administrative reasons. These reasons include the failure to pay the required registration fees. The Medical Act also gives doctors a right of appeal against decisions by the GMC to refuse to grant registration or a licence to practise or to withdraw registration or a licence to practise. Doctors who no longer wish to practise medicine can apply to the GMC for 'voluntary erasure' from the register.

The GMC maintains three registers:

- The register of medical practitioners – includes all doctors registered with the GMC
- The specialist register – includes the names of those doctors on the register of medical practitioners who are eligible to be appointed as consultants in the NHS
- The general practitioner register – includes the names of those doctors on the register of medical practitioners who are eligible to work as general practitioners in the NHS.

The GMC's legal powers for maintaining the specialist register and general practitioner register are not contained in the Medical Act but in a separate piece of legislation known as the PMETB Order.

Fitness to practise

The Medical Act gives the GMC powers and responsibilities for taking action when questions arise about a doctor's fitness to practise. The GMC relies on complaints and reports from enquiries before it initiates an investigation of a doctor. Following recent high profile cases, parliament, the media and the public no longer have confidence in this approach. Revalidation is being introduced as a proactive system requiring doctors to demonstrate that they are fit to practise.

The number of doctors about whom information received by the GMC led to a fitness to practise enquiry has steadily risen over the past 5 years. Approximately 80% of the referrals were from members of the public, with the remainder being made by someone acting in a public capacity. All enquiries are triaged within a week of receipt. Those that could never raise a question of impaired fitness to practise are closed without delay. Others proceed to either a further enquiry or a full investigation by trained medical and non-medical case examiners. The resultant outcome could be any one of the following:

- Referral to fitness to practise panel hearing
- Conclusion with advice
- Erasure
- Suspension
- Conditions
- Undertakings
- Warning
- Reprimand

- No impairment
- Voluntary erasure.

When it comes to a hearing, the function of the GMC as the regulator is not to strike off expensively trained doctors, but to try to ensure that they are safe to practise. The sanctions are necessary in the interest of patient safety and to preserve public trust in the profession.

Medical education

The GMC sets the standards for medical schools and medical students in its guidance *Tomorrow's Doctors* and conducts quality assurance visits to medical schools. The foundation programme is subject to standards and quality assurance that is jointly provided by the GMC and PMETB. The GMC is responsible for doctors in the first year of the foundation programme, who have provisional registration. The GMC publication *The New Doctor* sets out the standards that foundation programme providers must meet and the outcomes that these doctors must demonstrate before they are eligible to apply for full registration with a licence to practise. The GMC quality assures the foundation programme and conducts visits to Deaneries.

In February 2008 the government announced that PMETB would be merged with the GMC following a recommendation from Sir John Tooke's enquiry into 'Modernising Medical Careers'. The merger took place on 1 April 2010, enabling a seamless and continuous approach to medical education and training throughout doctors' careers. Providing a single point of responsibility from admission to medical school, through postgraduate training, to continued practice until retirement has helped to ensure consistency of expectations and standards.

Further reading

General Medical Council. http://www.gmc-uk.
  org (accessed 12 October 2010).

National Clinical Assessment Service

20

What is the National Clinical Assessment Service (NCAS)?

NCAS, previously the National Clinical Assessment Authority, was established as a special health authority in April 2001, following recommendations made in the Chief Medical Officer for England's reports, 'Supporting Doctors, Protecting Patients' (1999) and 'Assuring the Quality of Medical Practice: Implementing Supporting Doctors, Protecting Patients' (2001). In April 2005, the National Clinical Assessment Authority became the National Clinical Assessment Service, an operating division of the National Patient Safety Agency.

The support that NCAS provides can range from advice over the telephone, through more detailed and ongoing support, to a full assessment of the practitioner's performance. NCAS does not take on the role of an employer, nor does it function as a regulator. NCAS has offices in England, Northern Ireland, Scotland and Wales and provides its services to the whole of the UK, as well as Guernsey, Isle of Man and Jersey. It also provides services to the independent healthcare sector and the Surgeon General's Office.

Who does NCAS work with?

NCAS has developed working arrangements and in some cases 'Memoranda of Understanding' with a number of partners, including the GMC, General Dental Council, Healthcare Commission, health service ombudsman and the Academy of Medical Royal Colleges. These are designed to promote effective cooperation and allow for fast-track referral of cases as appropriate between the organizations. NCAS also works closely with the postgraduate deans, dentists', doctors' and pharmacists' representatives, patient bodies and other key stakeholders.

What does NCAS do?

NCAS helps to resolve concerns about the performance of dentists, doctors and pharmacists by providing confidential advice and support to healthcare organizations and to practitioners themselves. NCAS offers:

- Advice – from experts with backgrounds in clinical practice, healthcare and human resources management
- Specialist interventions – including facilitation, mediation, performance assessment, action planning and back-to-work support
- Shared learning – from case experience, evaluation and research, workshops and conferences.

Who will deal with the case?

There are three key groups of staff at NCAS who may be involved in handling a request for help: the casework team, advisers and assessors. The casework team has expertise in NCAS processes and procedures, and will manage the progress of the case. A member of the casework team will be the first point of contact at NCAS, taking the initial details about a request for help and passing the case to an NCAS adviser for more detailed advice. For support and assessment cases, a designated member of the casework team will be responsible for managing or supporting the progress of the case. The team provides either telephone or face-to-face advice on the local handling of these concerns.

The NCAS assessment

NCAS assessors undertake performance assessments in those cases where an assessment offers an appropriate way forward. The panel is always chaired by a lay member. NCAS has about 170 assessors, including lay assessors and clinical assessors from various specialties. All are trained in the use of NCAS assessment methods. In some of the smaller specialties, NCAS makes use of assessors directly nominated from the relevant Royal Colleges. Royal College assessors who assist in this way are always briefed on NCAS assessment procedures before undertaking the assessment.

The formal request for NCAS assessment is made by the chief executive of the employer or contracting body, or by senior managers acting formally on his/her behalf. They complete standardized documentation setting out their concerns. The referred practitioner is invited to offer comments. The assessment takes primarily a developmental rather than a pass/fail approach, and seeks to identify areas of satisfactory practice as well as areas requiring improvement. The assessment covers a range of aspects of practice, including clinical performance, behaviour and health.

An NCAS assessment is an intensive process for all involved. As part of the process of agreeing to an assessment, there is a meeting involving the NCAS case manager, the NCAS adviser, the practitioner and the employer or contracting body. The purpose of this meeting is to check that all parties understand the process and agree the way forward as proposed by NCAS. It is helpful for the practitioner to bring a friend or representative with them.

Following this, the assessment proceeds with three key components:

- Health assessment by an occupational health physician working with NCAS
- Behavioural assessment by a chartered psychologist with an occupational psychology perspective (one part-day and one full-day session, involving questionnaires and an interview). This element of the assessment looks at the practitioner's personal attributes and considers how these may be shaping their behaviour at work
- On-site clinical assessment (usually 2 days). The clinical assessors will be chosen from a field of practice as close to that of the practitioner as possible. Clinical performance is assessed with reference to relevant guidelines set by the regulatory body, college or faculty. Normally the clinical assessment will include a review of information provided by the practitioner and the employer or contracting body; a clinical record review; collection and consideration of views from colleagues and patients; direct observation of practice; review of the working environment; assessment of clinical decision-making; and an interview with the practitioner.

The assessment report is then drawn up over the following weeks. The findings will be listed and there will be recommendations both for the practitioner and the employer or contracting body. A draft report is sent out to the practitioner and the employer or contracting body for comments, which are then appended to the final report. The report may be shared with the appropriate postgraduate body in dentistry, medicine or pharmacy.

Suspension or exclusion

Sometimes performance concerns are so serious that they raise issues of patient safety and the question as to whether the exclusion of the practitioner is appropriate. NCAS has a role in helping to prevent inappropriate exclusion, and in trying to ensure that those cases which do proceed to exclusion are progressed fairly and as quickly and effectively as possible.

Support and remediation

Referral to NCAS, and in particular an assessment, could well be stressful for practitioners. The case manager and adviser ensure that practitioners are supported throughout the process. The *Back on Track* project was initiated by NCAS to create a national framework for remediation, re-skilling and rehabilitation programmes that enable practitioners to return to safe professional practice.

A list of NCAS good practice guidelines, as well as details of their conferences and educational workshops, can be found at www.ncas.npsa.nhs.uk (accessed 8 November 2010).

National Confidential Enquiry into Patient Outcome and Death

In 1982 a joint venture between surgical and anaesthetic specialties named the Confidential Enquiry into Peri-Operative Deaths (CEPOD) reviewed surgical and anaesthetic practice over 1 year in three regions in the UK. Subsequently in 1988 the National Confidential Enquiry into Peri-Operative Deaths (NCEPOD) was established supported by government funding and its first report was published in 1990. In 2002 NCEPOD extended its remit to include medical patients and changed its name to the National Confidential Enquiry into Patient Outcome and Death.

The remit of NCEPOD

NCEPOD undertakes confidential reviews of clinical practice and organizational care with the aim of improving patient care and safety. A qualitative peer review process that identifies both good practice and remedial factors in the delivery of care is used in all of its enquiries. When a study is completed, a report is published along with recommendations based on the findings of the enquiry.

How is NCEPOD governed and funded?

NCEPOD is independent of the Department of Health and the professional associations. It is both a charity and a company limited by guarantee. NCEPOD has a board of directors who are referred to as the NCEPOD Trustees. This board oversees the charitable and corporate governance of the organization. In addition, there is an NCEPOD Steering Group made up of nominated representatives of the various medical Royal Colleges and Associations and lay representation. There are also observers on the group from the National Patient Safety Agency (NPSA), the Coroners Society, the Institute of Healthcare Management, the Scottish Audit of Surgical Mortality and the National Institute for Health and Clinical Excellence. This board ensures the clinical integrity of the work that NCEPOD undertakes. Clinical input is provided by clinical coordinators who are practising consultants seconded from their NHS hospital.

NCEPOD is mainly funded by the NPSA. Financial support is also provided by the Health and Social Services Executive Northern Ireland, the offshore islands and the independent sector.

Study selection and analysis

Each year NCEPOD invites organizations or individuals to submit original study proposals for consideration as possible forthcoming studies. The proposals should be relevant to the current clinical environment and have the potential to contribute original work to the subject.

Once a study topic is selected, an expert group is formed to establish specific aims and objectives and design the relevant questionnaires. The latter are disseminated via a network of NCEPOD local reporters. The questionnaires are returned to NCEPOD where they are painstakingly anonymized and then confidentially peer reviewed by an advisory group of multidisciplinary healthcare professionals who reflect the clinical specialty mix for each study.

CPD accreditation for completing NCEPOD questionnaires

Consultants who complete NCEPOD questionnaires make a valuable contribution to the investigation of patient care. Completion of questionnaires also provides an opportunity for consultants to review their clinical management and undertake a period of personal reflection. These activities have a continuing medical and professional development value for individual consultants. Consequently, NCEPOD recommends that consultants who complete NCEPOD questionnaires keep a record of this activity, which can be included as evidence of internal/self-directed continuous professional development in their appraisal portfolio.

Current studies 2010/2011

- Surgery in children
- Perioperative care
- Cardiac arrest procedures.

Published reports

NCEPOD has published in excess of 28 reports looking at various aspects of clinical care, and many NCEPOD recommendations have shaped the way we practise and deliver healthcare in the UK. Each report is launched at a conference with active media engagement. Key healthcare professionals receive hard copies of these reports. Electronic copies are available via the NCEPOD website. Hospitals are also provided with a self-assessment tool that can be used to assess their compliance with the recommendations.

2010: Elective and Emergency Surgery in the Elderly: An age old problem
    Cosmetic Surgery: On the face of it
    Parenteral Nutrition: A mixed bag
2009: Deaths in Acute Hospitals: Caring to the end?
    Acute Kidney Injury: Adding insult to injury?
2008: Systemic Anti-cancer Therapy: For better for worse?
    CABG: The Heart of the Matter
    Sickle: A sickle crisis
2007: Emergency Admissions: A journey in the right direction?
    Trauma: Who cares?
2006: The Coroner's Autopsy: Do we deserve better?
2005: Abdominal Aortic Aneurysm: A service in need of surgery?
    An acute problem?
2004: Scoping our Practice
2003: Who Operates When – II?
2002: Functioning as a Team
2001: Changing the Way we Operate

2000: Then and Now
   Percutaneous Transluminal Coronary Angioplasty
   Interventional Vascular Radiology and Interventional Neurovascular Radiology
1999: Extremes of Age
1989–1996: Reports of NCEPOD

Examples of good practice that have developed from NCEPOD recommendations

- Local multidisciplinary audit meetings
- Peer review of mortality following operations
- Surgeons and anaesthetists no longer undertaking occasional paediatric practice
- Availability of 24-hour operating and recovery rooms in hospitals admitting emergency surgical patients
- Classification of interventions to assist organization and planning and to determine clinical priority – immediate, urgent, expedited and elective
- Uniform criteria and standards for both the investigation of reported deaths and the coroner's autopsy
- Emergency patients being seen by a consultant within a defined time limit
- Hospitals admitting emergency patients having access to 24-hour conventional radiology and CT scanning
- Organization of services and facilities for elective major vascular surgery.

Further reading

http://www.ncepod.org.uk (accessed 3
   November 2010).

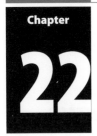

Chapter

22

National Institute for Health and Clinical Excellence

The National Institute for Health and Clinical Excellence (NICE) performs multiple roles: it provides guidance, sets quality standards and manages a national database to improve people's health and to prevent and treat ill health. It aims to produce high quality clinical guidelines with an independent open and transparent decision-making process, using the best available published evidence with input from experts and other interested parties.

NICE works with experts from wideranging fields, including the NHS, local authorities and many others in the public, private, voluntary and community sectors. It also places great emphasis on its 'Patient and Public Involvement Programme'.

Guidance

NICE produces guidance in three areas:

- Clinical practice guidelines – looking at new and existing medicines, treatments and procedures
- Public health – how to improve people's health and prevent illness and disease
- Health technologies – looking at new or existing treatments or procedures in the NHS.

Originally NICE established seven national collaborating centres (NCC) to develop its guidelines; however, following the merging of four there are now four national collaborating centres. Each collaborating centre is a partnership of professional medical and nursing organizations, e.g. the Royal Colleges, NHS trusts, academic units and patient/carer organizations. The NCCs are:

- The National Collaborating Centre for Women's and Children's Health
- The National Collaborating Centre for Mental Health
- The National Collaborating Centre for Cancer (NCC-C)
- National Clinical Guidelines Centre for Acute and Chronic Conditions.

NHS Evidence

NHS Evidence is a search engine that allows NHS staff to search the Internet for up-to-date evidence of effectiveness and examples of best practice in relation to health and social care. It was launched in 2009 to help manage the development and dissemination of knowledge in the NHS. The aim is to ensure that everyone working in health and social care has free, quick and easy access to quality assured, best practice information required to inform evidence-based decision-making. By using NHS Evidence an individual has access to more than 150 sources, including internationally respected evidence-based sources such as the Cochrane Library, the *British National Formulary* and the Map of Medicine.

In addition to providing web, medical database, journal and e-book searches, NHS Evidence is also home to more than 30 digital specialist collections, which provide annual evidence updates on key areas, giving a straightforward and succinct overview of what new research and evidence has been published.

NICE quality standards

In a major initiative, NICE is developing and defining the standards of healthcare that people can expect to receive for various major diseases. The aim of these standards is twofold: to provide information as to whether a specific treatment is clinically and cost-effective and whether or not it is viewed positively by patients.

The standards use the best available evidence from sources such as published NICE guidance and NHS Evidence. They are developed by NICE in partnership with the NHS and allied professionals and patients, and look at clinical effectiveness, patient safety and the patient experience.

NICE quality standards enable:

- Health and social care professionals to make decisions about care based on the latest evidence and best practice
- Patients to understand what service they can expect from their health and social care providers
- NHS trusts to examine the clinical performance of their organization quickly and easily, and assess the standards of care they provide
- Commissioners to be confident that the services they are providing are high quality and cost-effective.

Published NICE quality standards:

- Stroke
- Dementia
- Venous thromboembolism (VTE) prevention
- Specialist neonatal care.

NICE quality standards are currently being developed for the following topics:

- Depression
- Chronic obstructive pulmonary disease (COPD)
- Chronic kidney disease
- Diabetes
- Glaucoma
- End-of-life care
- Alcohol dependence
- Breast cancer
- Chronic heart failure.

Other NICE initiatives

- The NICE QOF Indicator Programme: a voluntary incentive scheme for GP practices in the UK, rewarding them for how well they care for patients using a points system

- The NICE Fellows and Scholars Programme, developed to contribute to the professional development of healthcare professionals and to encourage greater links between healthcare professionals and NICE
- The Scientific Advice Consultancy Service offers product-specific scientific advice to pharmaceutical companies and device manufacturers about products they have in development that may be referred for a technology appraisal
- The NICE International division: NICE International contributes to better health around the world through the more effective and equitable use of resources.

The future of NICE

Since 1999 NICE has made a huge impact on many aspects of healthcare. Since its inception it has developed new functions, expanded programmes and plays a central role in setting national standards. However, the exact role of NICE in the future has yet to be clarified and it seems likely that the coalition government will change this role. Initially it seemed that the role of NICE was set to be broadened with the publication of the White Paper 'Equity and Excellence: Liberating the NHS' in July 2010. However, there has been significant recent discussion in the medical media regarding the government announcement of a £200m cancer drugs fund which aims to allocate drugs to patients that are recommended by their doctors. This allocation would be regardless of the views of NICE and it is therefore perceived to undermine NICE.

Further reading

Maynard, A. and Bloor, K. (2010). The future role of NICE. *British Medical Journal*, **341**: c6286.

Collier, J. (2010). Drug pricing, NICE, and the PPRS: government gets it right. *British Medical Journal*, **341**: c6378.

http://www.nice.org.uk/aboutnice/ (accessed 19 December 2010).

Chapter 23

Postgraduate Medical Education and Training Board

The Postgraduate Medical Education and Training Board (PMETB) was an independent statutory body, responsible for overseeing and promoting the development of postgraduate medical education and training for all specialties, including general practice, across the UK. It assumed its statutory powers on 30 September 2005, taking over the responsibilities of the Specialist Training Authority (STA) and the Joint Committee on Postgraduate Training for General Practice (JCPTGP). PMETB was funded by grants from the Department of Health in England, Northern Ireland, Scotland and Wales. The board consisted of 29 members, with 17 medical representatives, eight lay members and four observers from the UK health departments. Appointments were made by the Secretary of State for Health. The board had two statutory committees – the Training Committee and the Assessment Committee.

PMETB's statutory responsibilities included establishing, promoting, developing and maintaining standards and requirements for postgraduate medical education and training across the UK. Its core functions were:

- Approving standards for assessments, trainers and training programmes submitted by medical Royal Colleges
- Monitoring training through inspection visits and other arrangements
- Awarding Certificates of Completion of Training (CCT)
- Determining eligibility of doctors for inclusion on the specialist and GP registers
- Setting the overarching principles under which selection into specialist training operate.

The Training Committee developed the standards, the curricula and the policy for quality assurance of postgraduate medical education. The Assessment Committee advised and made recommendations on all forms of assessment, including the levels of skill, knowledge, expertise and outcomes to be achieved in general practice and specialist training.

PMETB's remit did not extend to:

- Undergraduate medical education
- Recruitment and selection into postgraduate training programmes
- Workforce planning.

Merger of the GMC and PMETB

In February 2008, the government announced that the PMETB would be merged with the GMC, following a recommendation from Sir John Tooke's enquiry. This merger took place on 1 April 2010 with the GMC becoming the single organization responsible for the regulation of medical education and training at all stages of a doctor's career. All of PMETB's standards, processes and requirements have been adopted by the GMC.

GMC–PMETB and quality

Underpinning all of GMC–PMETB's work is an obligation to secure and maintain standards in postgraduate medical education and training in the UK. GMC–PMETB does this by monitoring training and outcomes through surveys and visits.

Approving curricula

GMC–PMETB works to ensure that curricula not only meet the standards for high quality training, but that they are consistent across all medical specialties in the UK. The standards are set out in the documents 'Generic Standards for Training and Standards for Curricula'.

Assessment

Each College that has received PMETB approval for a specialty curriculum is also required to submit an application for approval of the curriculum assessment system.

Consistency in training programmes – the PMETB visit

PMETB had a rolling visit programme of all Deaneries across the UK. These visits were informed by the 'Generic Standards for Training' and all included lay representatives.

Triggered visits

These were arranged in partnership with a medical Royal College, Deanery and others with training concerns. They were undertaken when there was serious educational failure which needed rapid investigation and where concerns could not be satisfied in any other way. These visits are likely to continue under the new structure.

Approving new training posts and programmes

A major component of GMC–PMETB's quality assurance work is being the sole competent authority responsible for the approval of posts and programmes. GMC–PMETB assesses each application and grants conditional or unconditional approval, taking into account the views of the Deanery and the College or Faculty.

National surveys

These surveys are designed to measure trainees' perceptions of their training and Deaneries are provided with reporting tools so that they can produce reports for a given specialty group at a given location. Deaneries can compare the perceptions of the trainees at the location against the perceptions of that specialty group nationally. GMC–PMETB also expect Deaneries to draw up action plans to address any concerns suggested by the surveys.

GMC–PMETB and certification

A major facet of GMC–PMETB's work is certifying doctors for application to the specialist and general practice registers. There are various routes to these registers, as outlined below.

CCT applications

A CCT is awarded to doctors who have successfully followed and completed a PMETB-approved curriculum in a PMETB-approved training programme. A CCT is a prerequisite for a doctor to work in the NHS as a general practitioner or substantive consultant.

CESR and CEGPR applications

GMC–PMETB manages a system that assesses applications from doctors who have not followed a traditional training programme but who may have gained the same level of skills and knowledge as CCT holders. These doctors can apply under Article 14(4) of the General and Specialist Medical Practice (Education, Training and Qualifications) Order 2003 for a Certificate confirming Eligibility for Specialist Registration (CESR) or, via Article 11 of the Order, for a Certificate confirming Eligibility for General Practice Registration (CEGPR). Applicants who have followed a career in academic medicine or undertaken training outside the UK in a specialty not recognized by GMC–PMETB can apply for a CESR under Article 14(5). Applicants applying by this route have to demonstrate that they have achieved the knowledge and skills consistent with practice as a consultant in the NHS.

GMC–PMETB and curriculum development

A key aspect of GMC–PMETB's mission is to ensure that the needs of tomorrow's patients, trainees and NHS are met. This is achieved through reviews of the content of curricula based on medical and social change, patient expectations, a changing workforce and service developments.

Chapter 24

Information management

Advances in information management and technology have made, and will continue to make, radical changes to the way healthcare is delivered. To work effectively in the NHS, a doctor must have an adequate and appropriate understanding of this area. This includes not only how to manage data and use technology, but also knowledge of its place in the organization and planning of the NHS. Doctors also need access to high quality information. This need has been recognized by independent inquiries and doctors' professional and defence organizations.

A modern IT infrastructure is vital to improving patient safety and enabling choice, helping clinicians to work efficiently and allowing them access to patient information promptly and securely. In 2002, Sir Derek Wanless, in his report on the English NHS, recommended doubling the IT budget and instituting a national programme for IT. He warned that without this 'the health service will find it increasingly difficult to deliver the efficient, high-quality service which the public will demand'.

National Programme for IT

The labour government made major investments in NHS IT, devising an ambitious national programme. The National Programme for IT (NPfIT), launched in 2002, is more extensive than any other IT programme in the world and represents the largest ever single IT investment in the UK. Critics have claimed that it is too centralized, too expensive and running late. In 2008, the National Audit Office reported that 'delivering NPfIT is proving to be an enormous challenge. All elements of the programme are advancing and some are complete, but the original timescales for the electronic care records service, one of the central elements of the programme, turned out to be unachievable, raised unrealistic expectations and put confidence in the programme at risk.' Nevertheless, it added that the 'original vision remains intact and still appears feasible'. By the end of 2009, many of the programme's systems and most of the infrastructure had been delivered successfully, with all acute trusts and 90% of primary care trusts having at least one system delivered through NPfIT.

The NPfIT infrastructure includes:

- The NHS Care Records Service (CRS) – connecting GPs and trusts in a single, secure national system; every patient will have a two-part electronic care record; the detailed care record will be formed from the detailed notes made by every healthcare professional treating the patient and will be held locally; a summary care record held nationally will contain essential information such as allergies and medication. A core data storage and messaging system, known as 'the spine' is central to the CRS (www.nhscarerecords.nhs.uk, accessed 28 December 2010)

- GP2GP, allowing electronic health records to be transferred between practices
- Choose and Book, the service enabling electronic booking for hospital appointments (www.chooseandbook.nhs.uk, accessed 28 December 2010)
- Electronic Prescriptions Service (EPS)
- A national Broadband IT network (N3) (www.n3.nhs.uk, accessed 28 December 2010)
- NHS Mail, a central email and directory service for the NHS
- NHS Web
- NHS Choices, the NHS online service for the public
- HealthSpace, a secure website where patients can store personal health information online (www.healthspace.nhs.uk, accessed 28 December 2010)
- Picture Archiving and Communications Systems (PACS) to capture, store, distribute and display digital medical images
- IT supporting GP payments, including the Quality Management and Analysis System.

NHS Connecting for Health

Connecting for Health (CFH) was set up in 2005 to support local NHS organizations in the planning, development and deployment of systems locally. CFH is delivering the NPfIT in England only. Scotland, Wales and Northern Ireland are developing their own IT programmes (www.connectingforhealth.nhs.uk, accessed 28 December 2010).

Security and confidentiality

The Caldicott report of 1997 made a number of recommendations for regulating the use and transfer of person-identifiable information between NHS organizations in England and non-NHS bodies. The recommendations of the Caldicott Committee defined the confidentiality agenda for NHS organizations. Central to the recommendations was the appointment in each NHS organization of a 'Guardian' to oversee the arrangements for the use and sharing of clinical information. A key recommendation of the Caldicott Committee was that every use or flow of patient-identifiable information should be regularly justified and routinely tested against the principles developed in the Caldicott report:

- Justify the purpose for using confidential information
- Only use it when absolutely necessary
- Use the minimum that is required
- Access should be on a strict need-to-know basis
- Everyone must understand his or her responsibilities
- Understand and comply with the law.

Since then developments in information management in the NHS have added a further dimension to the Caldicott role, e.g. the Data Protection Act (1998), the Human Rights Act (1998), the Freedom of Information Act (2000), the NHS Code of Practice on Confidentiality (2003), the inception of NHS Information Governance (2003), the election of the UK Caldicott Guardian Council (2005), establishment of the National Information Governance Board (2008), publication of the NHS Constitution (2009/10), etc.

Information and the law
Data Protection Act

This Act applies to all personal data and it places responsibility on data controllers (those responsible for the data) to manage it according to its principles. It is essential that personal data storage, whether on workplace or personal computers, conforms to the requirements of the Act. With the exception of anonymized information, most if not all NHS information concerning patients, whether held electronically or on paper, falls within the scope of the Act.

Freedom of Information Act

Information about public organizations is subject to the Freedom of Information Act. Therefore, all recorded information should be factual, to the point and information should be kept only as long as it is needed.

The Caldicott Guardian

It is important that the Guardian has the seniority and clear authority from the board/ senior management team, and the confidence of his or her colleagues. The Caldicott Guardian should play a key role in ensuring that the organization satisfies the highest practical standards for handling patient-identifiable information. The Guardian also has a strategic role that involves representing and championing information governance requirements and issues at board level. This role is particularly important in relation to the implementation of the NPfIT.

Key Caldicott responsibilities:

- Strategy and governance – champion confidentiality issues and act as both the 'conscience' of the organization and as an enabler for appropriate information sharing
- Confidentiality and data protection expertise – should develop knowledge of confidentiality and data protection matters
- Internal information processing – should ensure that confidentiality issues are appropriately reflected in organizational strategies, policies and working procedures for staff
- Information sharing – should oversee all arrangements, protocols and procedures where confidential patient information may be shared with external bodies.

Joint guidance on protecting electronic patient information

Everyone in the NHS has a responsibility to understand the implications of dealing with electronic patient data. The BMA and Connecting for Health have provided the following summary guidance to facilitate awareness of responsibilities.

The NHS Code of Confidentiality

Every individual is responsible for protecting patient information. Always log out of any computer system or application when work on it is finished; do not share logins with others and do not reveal passwords to others; change passwords at regular intervals; clear the screen of a previous patient's information before seeing another.

Organizational responsibilities

This includes organizational requirements for security, information governance and records management policies; completion of the information governance toolkit and statement of compliance, which measure and ensure progress against a series of standards; staff awareness of and training in good practice with regard to security.

NHS Connecting for Health's responsibilities

These include providing 'smartcards' and enabling legitimate relationships; setting up role-based access and facilitation of audit trails and alerts.

Chapter

25

Evidence-based medicine

Evidence-based medicine is the process of systematically finding, appraising and using contemporaneous research findings as the basis for clinical decisions (Rosenberg and Donald, 1995). Sometimes the term evidenced-based practice is used to reflect that the principles and practice can be applied in a wide variety of clinical situations.

The key steps in evidence-based medicine are:

- Developing the clinical question
- Searching the literature and identifying relevant articles and other resources relevant to the question
- Critically appraising the evidence to assess its validity and relevance
- Assessing the quality of evidence
- Applying the evidence.

One of the more controversial aspects of evidenced-based medicine is how to grade the quality of scientific evidence. Various systems are available to assess the quality of medical evidence, e.g. the US Preventive Services Task Force system, the National Health Service system, the Scottish Intercollegiate Guidelines Network system and the GRADE system (Grading of Recommendations Assessment, Development and Evaluation). The Scottish Intercollegiate Guidelines Network develops evidence-based clinical practice guidelines for the National Health Service in Scotland. It classifies levels of evidence as follows:

- 1++ High quality meta-analyses, systematic reviews of randomized controlled trials, or randomized controlled trials with a very low risk of bias
- 1+ Well conducted meta-analyses, systematic reviews, or randomized controlled trials with a low risk of bias
- 1− Meta-analyses, systematic reviews, or randomized controlled trials with a high risk of bias
- 2++ High quality systematic reviews of case control or cohort studies. High quality case control or cohort studies with a very low risk of confounding or bias and a high probability that the relationship is causal
- 2+ Well conducted case control or cohort studies with a low risk of confounding or bias and a moderate probability that the relationship is causal
- 2− Case control or cohort studies with a high risk of confounding or bias and a significant risk that the relationship is not causal
- 3 Non-analytical studies, e.g. case reports, case series
- 4 Expert opinion.

The GRADE system, the results of an international working party, provides a system for rating quality of evidence and strength of recommendations that is comprehensive and transparent. It is now recommended by several international organizations, and also publications such as the *British Medical Journal*, by the American College of Physicians and by the World Health Organization. GRADE classifies the quality of medical evidence into four levels:

- High quality – further research is very unlikely to change our confidence in the estimate of effect
- Moderate quality – further research is likely to have an important impact on our confidence in the estimate of effect and may change the estimate
- Low quality – further research is very likely to have an important impact on our confidence in the estimate of effect and is likely to change the estimate
- Very low quality – any estimate of effect is very uncertain.

Some organizations using GRADE combine the last two categories. The GRADE system offers two levels of recommendations: 'strong' or 'weak'. The strength of recommendation is based on the quality of the evidence and also on other features such as the acceptable or unacceptable effects of an intervention.

Advantages and disadvantages of evidence-based medicine

Evidenced-based practice clearly has the potential to improve the effectiveness of many diverse aspects of healthcare. It merges ongoing professional education and development with clinical practice. In this regard it is accessible for any grade of doctor. It can lead to greater uniformity of care locally and nationally and more effective use of resources.

However, evidenced-based practice also has its limitations. It can be extremely time-consuming searching multiple sources. The quality of recommendations may be limited by the quality of evidence available and this may be limited for various reasons, e.g. in some clinical situations it may be impossible or unethical to conduct a randomized controlled trial. Furthermore, the evidence available may only relate to one type of condition and it would potentially be erroneous to extrapolate that evidence to a variant of the same condition.

Reference and further reading

http://www.sign.ac.uk/pdf/sign50.pdf (accessed 18 January 2010).

Guyatt, G., Oxman, A.D., Vist, G.E. *et al.* (2008). Rating quality of evidence and strength of recommendations: GRADE: an emerging consensus on rating quality of evidence and strength of recommendations. *British Medical Journal*, **336**: 924–6.

Rosenberg, W. and Donald, A. (1995). Evidence based medicine: an approach to clinical problem-solving. *British Medical Journal*, **310**: 1122–6.

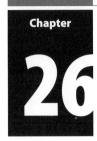

Research funding in the NHS

26

Alan Warnes

Introduction

The drive towards furthering knowledge in a clinical environment has been a motivator for those wishing to improve the healthcare of patients. Increasingly, new research requires peer review, ethical considerations and funding to support new initiatives, theories or hypotheses. This chapter provides information on funding for clinicians who wish to obtain support for their research.

At present there is a range of funding streams available to support clinical research; the recent introduction of the National Institute for Health Research has led to an additional sphere of relevant options, as part of the Department of Health funding initiative of £1025 million for 2010. These changes directed researchers towards obtaining competitive nationally peer-reviewed grant funding to support their research, through the NIHR or their recognized funding partners. Further funding is available through small charity organizations, industry and other agencies.

Support and development

Once a clinical investigator believes that there is potential in a new theory and has developed the basic outline of a protocol, he or she should arrange a meeting with the local Research and Development (R&D) Department to obtain their advice and support. The key factors that need to be considered for a successful grant application are:

- Protocol
- Collaborators (multidisciplinary team)
- Infrastructural support and facilities
- Intellectual property.

If support is not available through this mechanism, the Research Design Service (RDS) will be able to help. This is a newly established service whose prime directive is to help investigators generate sound grant proposals which will have the appropriate format, design and collaborators to help strengthen a research bid.

Protocol development may require further work depending on the experience of the investigator. This could include re-drafting the protocol so that it includes:

- A succinct title
- A summary, which should include a brief outline of the aims and objectives and how the study will be conducted
- Background, which should demonstrate how the proposed work or hypothesis fits in with current knowledge, obtained by systematic literature reviews
- Aims and objectives should be outlined which support the hypothesis

- Experimental design and methods, which should be able to demonstrate input from the patient population
- Data collection and management, including statistical analysis and health economic impact
- Study management, including a review of safety and ethical issues, highlighting any patient risks
- Resource requirements and robust costing analysis, outlining key issues which impact on the financial position of the study
- Study plan, which may include a flow chart of the study procedures (or a Gantt chart) and an appendix including all relevant supporting documentation (e.g. consent form, patient information sheet, questionnaires)
- Dissemination and outcome: how will the study's findings be made available and are there any implications for future practice and patient care?

Advice may also be needed on which funding body would be the most suitable to approach. The funding criteria are essential elements to consider prior to completing a research protocol, and the intended proposal needs to demonstrate how its activities, aims or objectives address the specifications of the funding call. This should include how organizational policies, systems, specialist treatments, staff, resources and good local practices support the request for financing.

Most grant applications require the support of a multidisciplinary team, of which statistical analysis, health economics and public and patient involvement are crucial. Inclusion of a clinical trials unit with pharmacy input is also essential when using an investigational medicinal product (IMP). The investigator may already be aware of suitable collaborators; however, if not, the local R&D department may be able to advise on the multidisciplinary support required. If essential collaborators cannot be identified, the RDS may be able to provide access to suitable partners. It is essential when considering collaborators to ensure that they have the appropriate background, skill set and experience to conduct the project activities.

It is also important to ensure that the appropriate facilities are in place for the proposed work to be carried out effectively. Successfully funded nationally peer-reviewed projects can be included on the NIHR portfolio, which confers membership to the NIHR faculty to researchers as long as part of their salary is included on the grant application. This can be as senior investigators, investigators, associates or trainees. Further, inclusion of projects on the portfolio also stimulates funding to the hosting or participating NHS trusts from the NIHR, which can be used to provide support for research services (e.g. research nurses, pharmacists, radiology, laboratory and pathology staff). Supporting infrastructure is a key element to developing successful grant applications.

The local R&D department can identify and protect any intellectual property, which may also impact on the type of funding required (e.g. NIHR i4i funding supporting innovative or high technology or business risk studies).

Funding bodies

The main types of funding bodies include:

- Department of Health: NIHR, Health Technology Assessment programme (HTA), Service Delivery Organization (SDO)
- Research Councils invest a combined sum of £2.8 billion in research across the full spectrum of academic disciplines, e.g. Medical Research Council (MRC) and Science Technology Foundation

- Major charities (Wellcome Trust, Cancer Research UK, British Heart Foundation)
- Local charities (which do not have national peer review mechanisms)
- Industry (with investigator lead proposals)
- EU Framework funding and USA National Institutes for Health (NIH) are also available but require strong collaborative links; preferable for established researchers.

The process for applying for funding through the majority of these organizations should be through their online systems or by contacting their helplines as each has their own registration mechanisms. The MRC, Cancer Research UK and Wellcome Trust all require pre-registration of the host organizations, which the researcher should check in advance of any applications. Also, each funding organization's requirements may differ, so investigators should plan their time to ensure applications are completed within the given timescales, especially to ensure that collaborators' contributions are included.

Management

Investigators need to ensure that appropriate procedures for effectively managing a successful grant award are in place via their employing organization or the organization receiving the grant. This should include:

- Probity and transparency – ensuring that funds are utilized according to the agreed terms and conditions of the financial contracts and that evidence of this can be provided
- Delivering the study plan – demonstrating the findings and results of the research
- Adherence to set timelines for pre-agreed milestones
- Progress reporting – the majority of funders will require expedited reporting on the progress of the research, which is usually on an annual basis
- Collaborations with external partners or services that may provide or take on certain project activities, e.g. monitoring, randomization, data analysis.

Funding calls

Please note that this chapter includes details of the major funding arms – there will be numerous calls from a range of organizations that are too numerous to mention. However, details of these can be accessed through web-based search systems. The most popular are the NIHR R&D information sites given below. These can be searched using a number of categories, which give contact links to the funding organization and details of the funding call.

Further reading

NIHR: http://www.nihr.ac.uk/Pages/default.aspx (accessed 20 October 2010).

http://www.nihr.ac.uk/infrastructure/Pages/infrastructure_research_design_services.aspx (accessed 20 October 2010).

http://www.nihr.ac.uk/faculty/Pages/default.aspx (accessed 20 October 2010).

http://www.nihr-ccf.org.uk/site/programmes/i4i/ (accessed 20 October 2010).

http://www.rcuk.ac.uk/default.htm (accessed 20 October 2010).

http://grants.nih.gov/grants/guide/ (accessed 20 October 2010).

http://www.rdinfo.org.uk/ (accessed 20 October 2010).

http://www.rdfunding.org.uk/ (accessed 20 October 2010).

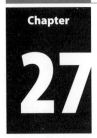

Research governance

Simon Lewis

Research is the key mechanism for the development and advancement of innovative medicines, clinical practice, exploratory treatments, novel therapies and healthcare delivery. The process of research is not isolated, but is governed by a range of legislations, policies, frameworks and directives, which are described in the Research Governance Framework (RGF, 2005). The RGF facilitates the national and legal standards for the conduct of research within the NHS, harmonizes the applicable regulations and ensures that the standards derived from this are implemented and maintained.

Research governance is needed to:

- Protect the wellbeing, health and safety of research participants
- Fortify accurate reporting, quality assurance and control
- Ensure the generation of reliable and valid data
- Ensure that research activities are ethical, legal and of good scientific quality
- Ensure that the appropriate liabilities and accountabilities are identified and put in place
- Promote pharmacovigilance to enhance reporting, reduce adverse events and protocol misconduct
- Encourage good clinical practice
- Ensure that research is monitored and audited, which supports both good clinical practice and the wellbeing of the patients.

The culminations of the various legislations have been transposed from the European directives into UK law as statutory instruments (http://www.opsi.gov.uk/, accessed 20 October 2010). It is important for any researcher to contact their own R&D department as soon as possible for guidance, as each organization has its own mechanisms to manage these fundamental principles.

Sponsorship and management

The RGF (2005) stipulates that a sponsor needs to be identified to take on the overall responsibility and management of a research project. This is usually undertaken by an organization, institute or company, which provides the appropriate levels of indemnity to cover any associated risks.

Sponsors may devolve key responsibilities for the conduct, monitoring and reporting to individuals, co-sponsors or subcontractors. This needs to be agreed and documented in a clinical trial agreement (www.ukcrc.org, accessed 20 October 2010). The delegation of tasks should reflect the intended research practices and be appropriate for the research to be undertaken.

Sponsors will always retain the overall liability for the research project; often the R&D department provides support for trust-sponsored projects and will also act on behalf of an investigator to recover any costs associated with the study, which are above standard clinical care.

Investigator responsibilities

Under the Medicine for Human Use (Clinical Trials) Regulations 2004 (SI No.1031), the investigator is defined as the authorized health professional responsible for the conduct of the trial at that site. If it is a team of professionals, the investigator is classed as the designated health professional leading the team.

Investigators in a multi-site study will consist of a chief investigator (CI) at the lead research site with research activities at participating trial sites delegated to a principal investigator (PI).

The primary responsibilities of an investigator are to ensure:

- That the research team are suitably trained and qualified to execute the research protocol
- Resources and facilities are adequate to support the research and it is feasible
- Documentation of the delegation of undertakings
- Provision of medical oversight and participant safety
- Adverse events are managed in line with protocol procedures
- Research is conducted in accordance with organizational policies and legal regulations, and that all the appropriate legal authorizations are in place
- The research team hold the appropriate substantive or honorary contracts with the host organization via a research passport or letter of access scheme (http://www.nihr.ac.uk/systems/pages/systems_research_passports.aspx, accessed 20 October 2010).

Research ethics

The involvement of research ethics committees (RECs) is to provide a favourable ethical opinion so that any research maintains the participants' rights, dignity and safety as subjected by the RGF and Clinical Trials Regulations 2004 (SI No. 1031).

To apply to an REC an investigator must submit study information via the Integrated Research Application System (IRAS) (www.myresearchproject.org.uk, accessed 20 October 2010). IRAS is a streamlined dataset which transfers research applications to the relevant regulatory bodies, such as the Medicines and Healthcare products Regulatory Agency (MHRA), for their approval.

Consent

The core component to ethical review is the consenting process. Arrangements for obtaining informed consent need to be proportionate to the type of investigation being conducted.

Consent is an ongoing process which should be informed and under no coercion. Potential research participants should be given options with no undue pressure to participate, nor should they feel the need to please their clinical care providers.

Clinicians acting as investigators must be confident that patients retain the study information and allow for appropriate discussions to ask questions and address concerns. The role of researcher should never impact on the role as clinician or affect duty of care.

The perceived patient benefit should always outweigh the potential risks (Declaration of Helsinki, 2008). Although patients may receive no direct benefit from participation, they must be aware of the associated risk and be given the opportunity to withdraw from the research project without having to provide an explanation and without their medical rights being affected.

In circumstances where the patient is unable to give informed consent through mental or physical incapacity, judgements need to be made as to the suitability to enter a patient into a project, and clinicians should work in accordance with the Mental Capacity Act 2005 and seek guidance from the RECs. The same measures should also be considered when recruiting vulnerable adults and children.

Regulatory approvals

Research involving the use of an investigational medicinal product (IMP), known as a clinical trial (CTIMP), has to seek authorization from the competent authority. In the UK this is the MHRA, and clinical trial authorizations (CTA) can be applied for through IRAS.

The governance surrounding clinical trials is very stringent, requiring management by committees, establishment of appropriate protocols, regular monitoring, regulatory inspections and safety reporting. Further guidance on clinical trials can be found at http://www.ct-toolkit.ac.uk/ (accessed 20 October 2010).

Depending on the research, other regulatory approvals can be sought through IRAS, including:

- National Information Governance Board (NIGB) providing exemption from taking consent
- Administration of Radioactive Substances Advisory Committee (ARSAC) additional exposure to radiation and radioactive materials
- Gene Therapy Advisory Committee (GTAC) for the use of embryos and stem cells.

CTIMPs must be conducted in accordance with the principles of Good Clinical Practice (SI No. 1928), which requires researchers to obtain specified accredited training in protocols, safety reporting and trial documentation.

The use of patient data must be clearly outlined and justified, subject to a favourable ethical opinion and must comply with applicable Caldicott principles (CP, 1997), organizational policies and the Data Protection Act 1998.

Research projects involving human tissue must have either a favourable ethical opinion with appropriate consent or an appropriate licence. This is often supported by material transfer arrangements to document the storage, collection and dignified disposal of samples in line with the Human Tissue Act 2004.

Trust R&D approval is the final authorization required before commencing research.

Summary

The regulations are in place to ensure that patient safety is paramount and that duty of care is a top priority in clinical research. This is supported by the investigators and sponsors working to good clinical practice and ensuring that all of their clinical responsibilities can be fully discharged.

Finally, clinicians wishing to undertake research need to ensure that potential risks and liabilities are proportionate to the intended activities, and they should utilize the RECs and R&D departments as key resources in gaining research approval.

References

CP. (1997). *Caldicott Principles 1997: Report on the Review of Patient-Identifiable Information.* http://www.dh.gov.uk/en/Publicationsandstatistics/Publications/PublicationsPolicyAndGuidance/DH_4068403 Department of Health (accessed 20 October 2010).

Declaration of Helsinki. (2008). *Ethical Principles for Medical Research Involving Human Subjects.* http://www.wma.net/en/30publications/10policies/b3/17c.pdf World Medical Association (accessed 20 October 2010).

DPA. (1998). *Data Protection Act 1998.* http://www.opsi.gov.uk/acts/acts1998/ukpga_19980029_en_1 Office of Public Sector Information (accessed 20 October 2010).

HTA. (2004). *Human Tissue Act 2004.* http://www.opsi.gov.uk/acts/acts2004/ukpga_20040030_en_1 Office of Public Sector Information (accessed 20 October 2010).

RGF. (2005). *Research Governance Framework for Health and Social Care,* 2nd edn. http://www.dh.gov.uk/en/Publicationsandstatistics/Publications/PublicationsPolicyAndGuidance/DH_4108962 Department of Health (accessed 20 October 2010).

SI No. 1031 (Statutory Instrument). *The Medicines for Human Use (Clinical Trials) Regulations 2004.* http://www.opsi.gov.uk/si/si2004/20041031.htm Office of Public Sector Information (accessed 20 October 2010).

SI No. 1928 (Statutory Instrument). *The Medicines for Human Use (Clinical Trials) Regulations 2004 (Amendment 2006).* http://www.opsi.gov.uk/si/si2006/20061928.htm Office of Public Sector Information (accessed 20 October 2010).

NHS financial flows

28

Introduction

The precise flows of money through the NHS are subject to regular review and change as different political leaders seek to obtain best value for the taxpayer.

The money spent by the NHS is public money, which is very different from private money in terms of the responsibilities placed on those that spend and those that audit the spend. There is a wealth of examples in history and from around the world of corruption in the use of public money. In the UK there are a multitude of processes to prevent corruption. These can seem to be impediments and to cause great frustration but are essential given the vast sums of taxpayers' money allocated to healthcare.

Where does the money come from?

Parliamentary vote

The government has an annual budget debated in parliament, which culminates in a vote to allocate a very large amount of money to the Department of Health to spend on the healthcare of the people.

The Department of Health budget

The Department of Health agrees with the Treasury how the budget will be spent. Traditionally a large proportion is distributed to the frontline via a capitation formula and a proportion is spent directly by the Department of Health. In the financial year 2009–10 the Department of Health spent £107bn on medical services, £1.9bn on public health and £0.8bn on health R&D, out of a total central government budget of £473.8bn.

Capitation formula

The majority of the budget is distributed locally to some form of commissioning agency, currently to primary care trusts (PCTs) on the basis of a weighted capitation formula. The allocation is based on the number of people living in a given area at the time of the last census with an adjustment for a number of factors such as deprivation index of the population, and any recognized population flows as evidenced by data on GP registration or primary school enrolment.

Commissioning

The principle in England has been that best value can be achieved by a commissioner/provider split where one organization has the funds and buys from, and holds to account, other organizations for the delivery of care.

This was introduced in the UK during the Thatcher government in the 1980s. Previously, different sections of the NHS were given budgets and had to accommodate as much clinical activity as possible within the centrally determined budget. There was no accountability and no incentive to strive to increase productivity. The then Conservative government introduced the concept of fund-holding in which GP practices who met certain criteria could hold the budget not merely for the patients' primary care but also for any necessary secondary care. The GPs negotiated and bought the required secondary care. Since a proportion of any savings accrued to their practice, there was a clear incentive to constrain access to expensive secondary care and to try to offer more services from within their practices.

The Labour government of 1997–2010 moved away from GPs controlling the budgets and created PCTs. These covered a population of 150 000–600 000. The PCTs commissioned care from hospitals and held the contracts with GPs. There was a phase during the early half of the Labour government when the focus was on increasing competition via an increase in types of provider. Private companies were encouraged to offer independent treatment centres, and contracts encouraged creation of 'any willing provider' status organizations that could compete with traditional NHS organizations. There were also some small attempts to encourage new providers to come into the GP market.

During this time, devolved administrations were created for Scotland, Wales and Northern Ireland. These administrations were given control over their health services and different structures evolved. The structures have created less of a division between the commissioners and providers, and are more subject to central control as opposed to market forces.

In the later part of the Labour administration there was some attempt to create practiced-based commissioning in which the funds for commissioning were devolved from the PCT to clusters of GPs. This did not become a reality in most areas. In practice, the PCT continued as the accountable body and spent most of its money on acute hospital care, mental health services, primary care, including contracts with GPs, and medication prescribed by the GP.

The coalition government elected in May 2010 has published a White Paper and associated documents which indicate their plans to give all the funds for care directly to GP consortia. These in turn will spend money on primary care services and commission secondary care. These organizations will be led by GPs.

The belief is that if the financial incentives in primary and secondary care can be aligned, then there is a possibility that extra effort will be exerted in provision of community services which in turn will save on the more expensive hospital services. There is some evidence to support this hypothesis from the Keiser Permanente experience in the USA. Implementation of this plan is in the early stages and will have to address many issues, not least of which is how medically qualified commissioners will balance their duty to cut cost with their duty to ensure safe and effective care.

Managing financial risk in commissioning

There is a recognition that, for some services (particularly for rarer problems), commissioning needs to cover a larger population. Traditionally, national specialist commissioning has been responsible for a limited number of services where there is a need for only one or two centres in the UK, and regional specialty commissioning has 'top sliced' funds from a number of PCTs to create budgets where there is a need for only one or two centres in any given region. There is often considerable history as to which services fall into these categories, but examples of services in these categories include services for cleft lip and palate, burns, HIV, etc.

Size of commissioning organization and financial risk

An example of this is the problem of Gaucher's disease. Enzyme replacement is the accepted treatment for a proportion of patients but this has a very high cost. Since the disease is inherited, the move of an affected family into the area covered by a commissioner carries a large cost. It is only in very large commissioning units covering many hundreds of thousands of patients that this additional cost can be easily absorbed into the day-to-day running costs.

Where does the commissioners' money go?

Most money is spent on purchasing care from acute and specialist hospitals, mental health services, general practice contracts, community medication and also the direct provision of community services. With the new requirements to separate commissioners and providers, it is likely that these community services will in future be independent or part of other providers.

Trust income

Trusts receive most of their income in relation to clinical services provided to local patients from a relatively small number of local commissioning units (PCTs or, in future, GP consortia). Other sources of income for trusts include specialty commissioning income, funding in relation to undergraduate teaching (traditionally termed SIFT – service increment for teaching), postgraduate education to cover the majority of the junior doctor salaries (previously termed MADEL – medical and dental educational levy), research and development (previously Culyer funding), in some cases income from private practice or other commercial opportunities such as rental of buildings or land.

The dilemma of commissioning

The commissioners have a fixed budget determined predominantly using a centrally set formula applied to the number of local people and their deprivation. This in turn allocates a slice of the nationally available funds to the commissioners. From this defined amount of money, all care has to be purchased. The expectation is that the requirement for care will be similar to that in the previous year. In practice, the demand for care and the costs of care owing to new technologies and general inflation have put pressure on the budgets to rise. Over the 60 years of the NHS this national allocation to healthcare has risen by 4–5% per annum, creating steady growth in the volume and quality of healthcare provision. The first dilemma is how does the healthcare system in the NHS adjust to the current predicted zero growth or possible contraction. The second dilemma is what happens if the year-on-year demand is not similar, but in fact demand rises at, say, 10% per annum. The commissioners' budgets are fixed, but the costs of care rise in relation to the increased provision. This leads to a crisis and various attempts to reduce demand termed 'demand management'.

GP income

GPs are independent subcontractors whose businesses receive funding predominantly from their local commissioners, in part in relation to capitation (number of patients registered with the practice) and in part in relation to specific arrangements for service delivery, which have recently been linked to the delivery of certain quality standards in the quality and outcomes framework (QOF).

Where does money go in a trust?

At the start of the financial year the trust has been given an expectation of what work it will be required to do and an indication of the associated income. This is converted into an annual budget, which is then broken down to individual departments. In practice, the departmental budget is usually similar to the previous year but with modifications to suit changing patient flows or agreed service developments.

The majority of the money is spent on the clinical frontline services with a proportion for the corporate services such as finance, HR, IT, cleaning and maintenance. Approximately 6% is spent on the buildings, either as a repayment on a loan as in a PFI scheme, or as public capital dividend, which is money given back to the Department of Health in essence as rental for the hospital buildings. On aggregate, 60–65% of the money in a hospital is spent on staff salaries, around 30% on consumables and the rest on the buildings.

The experience curve, Gershon savings and unfunded service developments

An important issue is the Gershon efficiency savings. In any normal commercial business, companies that have greater experience or produce more of a product become better at doing the work or making the product, and this is reflected in greater efficiency and lower cost. A graph can be drawn of cost per unit of production against volume of production and this 'experience curve' exhibits progressive cost reduction in relation to volume of production. A review by Gershon created a formal requirement on government departments and public sector organizations to do likewise. A minimum of a 2.5% reduction per annum on all budgets is imposed to reflect the presumed growth in efficiency with experience. The process for funding the introduction of new drugs, other technologies, or novel more expensive ways of assessing or treating patients has to be funded outside the normal process of rolling forward the annual budgets. New developments can only be funded by fully costed business cases which identify new income. A regular problem occurs when medical staff grow a service or introduce new technology without going through the process of a business case and identifying new funding. There is never enough money in existing budgets which reduce by 2.5% per annum to cope with the costs of the service developments. These unfunded service developments are a source of considerable friction between consultants and managers.

Demand management

In a state-funded system with a limited budget, the problem is how to limit demand for healthcare to match the budget. If this fails, then unacceptable waiting lists start to build up as the number of patients arriving within any time period exceeds the funds available to deliver care. Methods to achieve demand management have included: financial incentives, for example within GP fund-holding, to create primary care alternatives to hospital referral; create checking systems on referrals; use nurse or physiotherapist triage; limit availability of certain categories of treatment (e.g. via NICE or Local Priority Setting Committees); limit access to low priority procedures and to create alternative low cost community provision, e.g. community matrons. These have all had variable success.

Devolved administrations – Scotland, Wales and Northern Ireland

The devolved administrations have progressively differing arrangements to England for funding and organizing healthcare. An important point is that these areas receive from central government under the Barnett formula £1.20 to spend on healthcare for every £1 spent in England.

Chapter

29

The contract

Those responsible for buying care on behalf of the community, the commissioners, follow Department of Health guidance in drawing up a contract for the care to be delivered. The providers have to satisfy the contract. There are inherent tensions in this, since demand for care from the population may exceed the commissioners' budget and clinicians want to introduce new approaches which may not be on the commissioners' priority list.

The financial agreement

Each year in the autumn, commissioners and trusts discuss anticipated activity and possible new service developments for the forthcoming financial year. By midwinter a detailed contract has been written and the trusts are expected to sign their agreement to the contract. This drives the internal budget of the provider and over the financial year there are regular contract monitoring meetings to ensure that delivery occurs.

Block contract

Traditionally the agreement was based on delivering the same care as the previous year, with perhaps an uplift in funding to take into account specific issues such as the cost of specific new drugs or anticipated rise in the cost of blood or centrally determined pay rises. All activity then had to be accommodated with the funding of this block contract.

Tolerances – collar and cap

The next level of sophistication allowed a certain flexibility in the funding according to the number of patients in different categories, but with absolute limits on the minimum and maximum amount of money a trust would receive, sometimes termed a collar and cap. This created a degree of risk-sharing since the commissioners would not overspend if the volumes went up and conversely the trust covered the fixed costs even if few patients arrived.

Payment by results (PbR)

In a normal business, money would follow patients and the more patients came to the trust, the more money the trust would receive. This has been tried, but in circumstances where demand grows and outstrips the budget of the commissioners, then in practice an agreement has to be reached on a maximum payment of funds to the trust irrespective of the number of patients. This leads to the concept of over-performance.

Over-performance

Suppose the contract anticipates 1000 patients of a particular type per annum, but in fact local GPs refer 1100 – this exceeds the commissioners' budget but the trust has incurred real cost in treating these patients. In fact, since the trust had not anticipated this work and has not employed sufficient staff for the extra 100 cases, high cost locums may have been needed, so the cost of caring for the extra 10% of patients may in fact constitute a 15% increase in cost. The counter-argument is that since the buildings and most of the staff are already there, then the additional cost should be lower and reimbursements should be at a lower 'marginal' rate. This was highlighted in the 2010–11 national requirement on hospitals to receive only 30% of the tariff for emergency cases exceeding the number treated in 2008–09. This area is particularly difficult for trusts.

Demand management

To address this, the NHS has adopted a variety of methods to contain the numbers of patients treated by hospitals. One approach is to keep people waiting. Latterly more sophisticated approaches have been tried, such as triaging patients to identify those who can be treated by lower cost alternatives to hospital care.

Activity targets

Typically the contract will reinforce government policy by imposing financial penalties for failing specific government targets, such as seeing 98% or 95% of patients attending A&E within 4 hours or ensuring that all elective patients have received their care within 18 weeks.

Data

The success of the contract with all parties rests on accuracy of the data. This in turn relies on coding and the coders being able to glean the correct information quickly and accurately from the clinical records. Commonly there are disputes between commissioners and the trust which may be manifest as data challenges and require great resources to be directed at proving what happened to patients and that the action was indeed necessary, and not a result of a subtle change in clinical practice driven by the incentive of increasing income.

Quality and the contract – CQUINS

The 2009–10 contract introduced the idea that the commissioners would hold back funds from their budget and use these as incentives to deliver desired quality outcomes. These quality and innovations (CQUINS) have increased in value. They include nationally, regionally and locally set quality targets. To date they seem to have focused on desirable evidence-based clinical benefits such as ensuring that patients admitted to hospital are assessed for the risk of venous thromboembolism.

In the USA this area is well developed, with the concept of pay for performance. The quality indicators include achieving patterns of drug prescribing and achieving compliance with care bundles.

Gershon savings

Any business should become more efficient with experience. In commercial business an experience curve can be drawn to show the reduction in unit cost of production against total cumulative volume of production. The same logic has been applied to public sector services and in 2004–05 Sir Peter Gershon recommended that all budgets reduce by 2.5% per year. New services or service developments in the year need new budget allocations over and above this reduction. Thus the core contract with the commissioner will reduce in amount year on year, and then money will be added on for central cost pressures or new developments.

Central cost pressures

These are costs that the healthcare system has to bear which have been introduced by central government without any discretion to the local health economy. These include the results of national pay bargaining with the unions or nationally agreed increases in the price of consumables such as blood or NICE-approved new drugs or an increase in premium paid to the National Health Service Litigation Authority (NHSLA) for medical indemnity.

Service developments

Medical staff understandably want to introduce the latest approaches to managing their patients. This normally costs money and constitutes a service development. To fund these developments the trust has either to find a compensatory saving or persuade the commissioner (by around September of the year before the change is to be introduced) that the cost needs to be covered in the following year's allocation.

Growing the service and unfunded service developments

Consultants rightly want to build their clinical practice. However, they commonly feel frustrated by this budget process and introduce a new technology or grow the service outside of the budgetary allocation process. This inevitably results in an overspend and a great deal of stress, if the service then has to be withdrawn or reduced in scale.

SIFT, R&D, MADEL

Trusts can receive three other income streams indirectly from central government.

The service increment for teaching (SIFT) is given in relation to undergraduate teaching. There is a fixed component and a variable component, which relates to student numbers. There is considerable argument about the correct proportion of these elements and there may be some changes over the next year or so.

There have been a number of changes over the past 5 years in the funding that trusts receive to support R&D. Currently the funding is moving towards a system where trusts are essentially reimbursed in relation to the number of patients entered into nationally approved trials. This process is managed by the comprehensive local research network and a process must be followed to enrol a trial onto the list of approved studies.

The postgraduate medical and dental education levy (MADEL) is a stream of funding which pays for the salaries of junior staff and supports the postgraduate education department. It is also changing from a centrally controlled Deanery budget to a devolved budget held by local commissioners who essentially buy training from local providers.

Specialty commissioning

Some trusts offer services for relatively rare conditions where large populations are required to generate sufficient volumes of patients. Examples include cleft lip and palate surgery, burns, etc. These cannot be commissioned by small local organizations and are addressed through specialty commissioning.

Private practice

Some trusts have the ability to earn considerable income from supporting the delivery of private practice. Many of these trusts have been financially strong and have achieved foundation status. Originally, foundation status limited the proportion of their income that could be derived from private practice. This limit has now been lifted.

Other – interest, rental, etc.

Some trusts earn from renting space to retailers or cafés, and others have other generally minor income streams such as bank interest.

Prioritization

When demand exceeds the budget, some prioritization decisions have to be made which carry the support of the community and do not breach regulations such as the Human Rights Act. At a national level, NICE takes on this task. At local levels most commissioners have the support of some sort of prioritization committee. This will identify low priority procedures such as many cosmetic surgical procedures which will not be funded. There will typically be some procedures where funding will only be provided if certain stipulations are met in terms of pre-assessment for complications or if delivered under strict protocols in a limited number of centres. There is usually an appeals process for individual patients who believe their case constitutes an exception to the general rule. Consultants are often invited to participate in these committees to ensure that specialist expertise is included in the deliberations.

The contract is also guided by the desire to reduce duplication and follows the national policy of moving care from hospitals to community settings, for example by reducing the number of outpatient follow up appointments. It is likely that over the next few years the quality, innovation, productivity and prevention (QIPP) agenda will also drive the contracts.

30 The quality, innovation, productivity and prevention (QIPP) agenda

In the face of public sector cutbacks there is a drive to improve efficiency but not at the expense of quality. A number of national work streams have been initiated to drive this forward. This approach, when combined with service targets, has been very effective at cutting hospital-acquired infection by MRSA and *Clostridium difficile*. The national work streams fit into three key areas: commissioning, provider efficiency and system enablers.

Commissioning

- Safe care – will cut pressure ulcers, catheter-acquired urinary tract infections and falls
- Right care – will focus commissioning on high value, whole system pathways and networks rather than institutions. A key is the analysis of unexplained variations in spend on healthcare and health outcomes for the commissioners' population
- Long-term conditions – target management of those at risk to prevent disease progression, maximizing self-management, providing joined up and personal services and workforce development
- Urgent care – seeks a 10% reduction in the number of patients attending accident and emergency
- End-of-life care – aims to improve provision of services and management of the cohort of end-of-life patients.

Provider efficiency

- Back office efficiency – improved use of non-clinical resources
- Procurement – better value central purchasing
- Clinical support – centralization of some services such as pathology (following the Carter report), application of lean processes
- Productive care – ensure best practice in productivity is spread across English hospitals
- Medicines use and procurement – optimizing value for money on medication spend.

System enablers

- Primary care contracting and primary care commissioning – examine how the GP contract can support the wider QIPP agenda
- Technology and digital vision – support in the development of regional and local IT strategy.

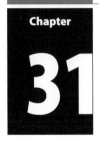

The budget

The budget is the amount of money handed to each department to allow it to deliver the business plan. The budget is a tool for control since monthly underspend or overspend identifies that the plan is not being followed.

The budget cycle

In an ideal world the contract is agreed before Christmas. The business plans are determined in January and the budgets for each part of the organization signed off before the end of February in time for the Board to agree them in March before the start of the financial year.

What does the budget look like?

The budget is usually divided by month. There is a pay element to cover salaries and a non-pay element to cover consumables. Commonly the budget is the amount of money given to a department the previous year with some percentage increase to take into account nationally agreed salary increases or other national cost pressures, and some specific uplift to fund specific agreed service developments. Each element of pay and non-pay is broken down to the funding required for specific posts and for specific categories of consumables.

Managing peaks and troughs

Some fluctuation in spend can be predicted in line with Christmas and summer holidays and winter pressure from emergencies. These should even out across the year, but some organizations take these into account in providing a budget.

Why does the budget always seem wrong?

The budget is never wrong. It is the money allocated to the department. The problem is that the detail may not match what is happening on the ground. Over time small decisions are made which change how the money is spent. One full-timer is replaced by two part-timers, or a person is employed to save a threatened income stream. These changes accumulate. Every so often, it is essential to look at the detail again and re-align the spend with the money allocated in the budget.

Activity planning

Key to successful management of the budget is the activity plan. The number and type of patients anticipated to be seen determines the staffing requirement and the projected consumable use.

'Unfunded beds'

Unfunded beds are created when activity planning goes wrong. If there are more patients in the hospital than can be afforded by the budget, safe care requires that the patients are cared for but the salaries and consumables are paid for outside the budget. This will create an overspend. It may be that this unanticipated number of patients will attract additional income or that the trust will create a deficit.

Service line reporting

Service line reporting ensures that each service understands the income it receives each month and the costs incurred by their service either directly or indirectly in other departments such as imaging, pathology or pharmacy. Departments should make at least a 20% surplus so that there is money to pay for corporate infrastructure (heating, lighting, rates, etc.) and to provide funds to invest in new equipment and service developments. The surplus after the corporate overheads have been paid is the earnings before interest, tax, depreciation and amortization (EBITDA). Amortization is depreciation in intangible assets.

EBITDA

EBITDA reflects the money made by the operating part of any business. It is a measure of operating efficiency. When expressed as a percentage of turnover, EBITDA is used by the regulatory organization Monitor to regulate foundation trusts.

Ratio analysis

To try to enhance the understanding of the efficiency of the business, ratios such as income per full-time equivalent employee or profit per full-time equivalent are used in a similar way to those seen in commercial company accounts.

Costs

Patient level costing

Patient level costing is a further development where the income and costs of each patient are understood. This allows individual clinicians to understand when clinical management plans are likely to cost more than the associated income.

Variable versus fixed costs

Simplistically, it might seem that there should be a direct relationship between the number of patients seen and the cost to the organization. However, there is a considerable fixed cost that has to be paid just to be in the business of seeing patients. This covers equipment and the salaries of the team. Often in healthcare the cost for each additional patient seen (termed marginal cost) is relatively modest and is accounted for by the consumables used by each patient.

Step costs

At some point, as the number of patients increases the capacity of the fixed costs to accommodate more patients becomes limiting and there is a step in the costs if there are further increases in patient numbers to be treated. For example, an additional consultant may need to be employed.

Cutting costs

Every year every trust has a cost improvement plan (CIP) to respond to Gershon savings. Standard approaches include:

- Review procurement to seek better value contracts with suppliers
- Review drug expenditure to reduce use of high cost drugs
- Consolidate duplicate services
- Close unfunded beds
- Try to smooth variation in patient flows so that additional staff are not required to deal with surges
- Re-profile elective activity to make space for predictable surges such as winter pressures
- Agree common clinical protocols so that a limited range of consumables can be used and less expensive staff can provide a greater proportion of the care.

Chapter

32

Writing a business plan

The business plan or business case is the template on which all investment decisions are made, whether the investment involves one-off capital or a stream of future funding to support salaries and consumables. The document is the justification for spending the taxpayer's money on a project and needs to weigh up the objectives/benefits against the estimated costs and risks.

The scale can vary from tens of thousands of pounds to billions when commissioning a new hospital. Very large cases tend to be divided into stages with a strategic outline case and then a full business case. Both of these have set structures and requirements.

Background

A standard internal business case has a number of sections and has to answer a number of questions:

- What is the problem you want to solve?
- What is the scale of the impact of the problem?
- How do the issues fit into the organizational strategy?
- Is this a department in which to invest?

The Executive will need a succinct summary of the problem and its impact on the organization. The organization will have a strategy. It will have a plan to grow certain services and not others. There will be a view on the importance of certain activities in the context of government targets and commissioner intentions. You will have to explain how your proposal is in harmony with this strategic plan if it is to succeed.

Monitor recommends that services are examined for their contribution to the fixed costs of the organization. The idea is that those that make the greatest contribution justify further investment, whereas those that cost more than they earn should be examined for cost reduction rather than investment. Where is your department in terms of profitability?

The 'do nothing' option

- Why can't you leave the problem alone?
- What are the patient care, regulatory and financial implications of doing nothing?
- Why has this risen to the top of your priority list?

The default position has to be to do nothing. The organization has only limited resources. Many areas are crying out for investment. Why not leave this problem alone and go and spend whatever money there is on a higher priority. It has to be very clear to the Executive why the 'do nothing' option is unsustainable. Good examples are health and safety or fire risk. If an external organization has issued an instruction on the basis of safety, the status quo is clearly untenable.

Benefits

- What benefits are you hoping to achieve – clinical, financial, reputational, regulatory?

This has to be really clear. How will the service look once the investment is made? Can you put some numbers to this? For example, if the investment is to support the enhanced recovery programme, what is the current length of stay for the operations upon which you are focusing? What is the future anticipated length of stay? How many patients will benefit? What does this mean in terms of bed days saved? What will you do with these saved beds? Will you close a ward? What cash savings will be derived? What is the patient feedback like currently? How will the proposal resolve any consistent problems identified in the feedback? What about clinical quality issues and patient safety incidents – how will the proposal impact on existing data in these areas?

Options

- What solutions have you examined?

You need to have looked at several different ways of solving the problem, not just your favoured one. If you cannot think of more than one solution, ask someone, see how others round the UK or even other countries have addressed the same problem. Think outside the box. The Executive will push you to have explored a range of options which cut cost. From this, you need a short list.

- For each solution what will you do?
- How will it deliver the benefits?
- Will all the benefits be delivered?

You can expect to be pressed on the detail of how the patient pathway will look for each option, especially the preferred option. You need to know what different tasks will be required of staff. You need to have a plan for staff training.

What is the timescale?

Over the months ahead, on what dates do the costs, benefits and income start coming in? Typically this is very different for the different options.

What new income will be generated and when will this come on stream?

Money to pay for the investment has to come from somewhere. So understanding the associated income stream and when it arrives is very important.

How would service delivery change and what cost reductions would be obtained from that change?

This is a real opportunity to strengthen the case. The Executive are going to be much more interested in investments which redesign clinical services to improve the patient experience, reduce the number of steps and reduce the number of staff. Typically this is where IT business cases fall down in that everyone can see that the investment will improve the delivery of service – however, without a radical change in the clinical process, it is unclear which posts will be closed to pay for the ongoing software licence.

What will it cost in both capital and revenue and when will these costs come in?

You will need help from the finance department for this section. Capital costs are treated separately from ongoing revenue costs. The organization agrees a capital budget at the beginning of the year. It will be important to plan in which year all or part of the capital will be spent. Any VAT implications will be important. Revenue costs will need to include salaries, software licences and the costs of new consumables. The supplier may be offering lease or buy deals. There may also be hidden costs where the supplier discounts the equipment knowing that they can recoup the money by being a monopoly supplier of high cost consumables.

When obtaining quotes from suppliers, you need to remember that you cannot enter into any obligation with a supplier and that the quotes are only indicative. If you are successful you will have to go to competitive tender for the provision of any external product or service. You need to be very careful about developing any relationship with suppliers as this may prejudice your position as a judge in a subsequent tendering process.

In big projects which take years to come to fruition, it can be difficult comparing the value of projects when the costs are incurred at different times, and the income streams also come in at different times. There is a mathematical tool called 'Net Present Value' which is used to convert all future income and costs streams into what would be the net value today.

Risk – what could go wrong?

- Will it work? What are the risks that it will not solve the problem? What are the risks that the implementation will fail?
- How will you mitigate these risks?
- How much will this mitigation cost?

Change is difficult. Many things fail. Make a list of all the things that are outside your control and which could happen that would result in this project failing to deliver the benefits. For example, if you work in a small town and need to recruit specialized staff, how likely is it that there will be any available to recruit? For each of the risks how do you score them: high/medium/low?

If you want to quantify the risks more thoroughly, can you give the chance of each risk happening a mathematical P value? In the next column write down what you would do if it happened, and in the next what it will cost to respond to the risk. Finally, in the last column multiply the P value by the cost of mitigation. This gives an 'expected' financial value for each risk.

One of my non-executive directors used to ask the Executive 'If you personally had to take a 25% cut in salary if this investment made a loss, would you do it?'

Consultation

Consult relevant stakeholders (other service leads, patients, external agencies) and review in the light of their comments. If your proposal requires another department to work differently or make some investment in time or equipment, you will need written confirm-ation that they have agreed to this. A frequent problem arises when a surgical specialty has a requirement to appoint a new post, perhaps as a result of a Deanery criticism of training, and the authors forget the cost implications of appointing a consultant surgeon to the anaesthetics or pathology department. If your case requires the commissioners to provide a new income stream, you need written confirmation that this will be forthcoming.

Construct a chart summarizing the analysis of the business case

Typically the document ends with a chart giving as a minimum: column 1, the options (including 'do nothing'); column 2, relative score/assessment for delivering benefits; column 3, relative score for risks; column 4, net financial cost; column 5, ranking.

Produce a preferred option

You need to make a specific recommendation to the Executive which will be accepted or rejected.

How to create a winning business case

Finally, write it up using the format used by the Executive in your organization for business cases and keep it short. It is all too easy to have a 'data-dump' when writing a business case. This just leaves everyone confused. Craft the case so that all the information is there in well chosen succinct form. Use graphs and pie charts as well as financial tables. Discuss with some of the members of the Executive so that they are well briefed. Remember, you must submit the document prior to the deadline for the circulation of the papers to the meeting at which you wish the decision to be made.

Chapter 33

NHS structure and organization

Organization and reorganization

The NHS is over 60 years old and has experienced many reorganizations. The satirical Roman author Gaius Petronius wrote 'We trained very hard, but it seemed that every time we were beginning to form up into teams, we would be re-organised. I was to learn later in life that we tend to meet any new situation by re-organising, a wonderful method of creating the illusion of progress while producing inefficiency and demoralisation.'

Recurrent reorganizations in the NHS try to address the following tensions:

- The market versus central budgets – how can the service be made both more responsive to patient needs, deliver better value for money and yet offer an integrated service?
- Employment of staff versus outsourcing – can one manage a group of staff better by direct line management or via a contract with an independent company which has to deliver to stand a chance of keeping the contract?
- National accountability versus responsiveness to local needs – the NHS was conceived as a national service. Aneurin Bevan famously said that 'If the bedpan lands on the floor in the hospital in Tredegar, I want the noise to reverberate through the corridors of Westminster'. There is a view that all citizens should have equitable access to the full range of services and that one's postcode should not determine the nature of the services available. Conversely, different parts of the country have different profiles of needs and different patient groups lobby for different investments.
- Capital financing – very expensive projects such as building a new hospital constitute a major drain on exchequer funds. How can the private sector use its capital to fund the build and be reimbursed over time by the government?
- Growth in spend – how can the government cope with both growth in demand for health services and the annual rise in new medical and equipment costs?
- Growth in public expectation – owing to improved standards of living, exposure to more information on what is available around the world and on the quality outcomes from British healthcare, there is a rising expectation of what healthcare should be provided.
- Voter power – the NHS employs more than 1 in 20 British voters.
- Aligning incentives – different configurations confer different incentives and behaviours. Kaiser Permanente, a California-based health service provider, offers high quality care and has many similarities to the NHS. One of the reasons that it is able to deliver very good value for money is the integration between primary and secondary care such that the incentives of both are aligned. Thus the service can make a trade-off in expenditure based on appropriateness and cost-effectiveness rather than artificial budget categories.

England

The structure of the NHS proposed by the coalition government is in development but seems to involve a number of layers:

- Department of Health – this will be responsible for policy but not day-to-day decision-making. The size of the department will be reduced
- Three groups report directly to the department with responsibility for the day-to-day running of the NHS:
  - The NHS Commissioning Board – this will oversee GP consortia, undertake direct commissioning in some areas such as maternity services and set national priorities and outcomes
  - Care Quality Commission – this will regulate the quality of all organizations that offer healthcare, by setting standards and giving a licence to organizations on the basis of meeting the core standards
  - Monitor – this will be the economic regulator for all NHS-owned hospitals which will become foundation trusts
- GP consortia – these consortia will be responsible for commissioning care for perhaps 500 000 people and will comprise GP leaders appointed from the different localities covering this population. The consortia will commission care from hospitals and will be encouraged to shop around to achieve best value and outcomes
- Patients and public will be encouraged to exercise choice based on much more open information on quality of services and outcomes
- HealthWatch, a new patient watchdog agency, will be created to give patients and their interests a clear voice
- The Department of Health will be supported by a reduced number of arm's-length bodies addressing specific regulatory functions.

The coalition government proposals are set to replace a system where the Department of Health was intimately connected to day-to-day delivery and where, for one period, the posts of chief executive of the NHS and the Permanent Secretary of the Department of Health were held by the same individual, Sir Nigel Crisp. Regional strategic health authorities reported to the chief executive of the NHS. These in turn exerted authority over primary care trusts (PCTs) and the provider organizations. The PCTs commissioned services from acute trusts and paid for services from GPs. They also often directly employed a number of nursing and therapy services. Some of the providers were foundation trusts and enjoyed a varying degree of greater independence. Monitor regulated the foundation trusts and the Care Quality Commission monitored quality of all the provider organizations.

The providers of NHS services

There are many people who believe that the NHS should remain 'public'. In practice it is not so simple to decide what 'public' means.

The largest numbers of patients seen daily are those who attend general practices, many of which are owned by individuals or partnerships of GPs. Traditionally, hospitals have been owned by the government. Over the past decade many patients have received care, particularly surgery, at independent sector or private hospitals with the care paid for by the NHS.

This is likely to increase. Some private organizations have taken over the management of NHS hospitals, as is the case with Hinchingbrooke hospital, which is to be run by 'Circle'. The coalition has indicated a desire to encourage other models such as Social Enterprise. This is likened to the ownership structure of John Lewis plc. The Central Surrey Health providers of nursing and therapy services are the prime NHS example. The organization essentially left the NHS and has a model where the organization is owned by the employees but is not-for-profit, ploughing back profits into the development of services. This is a successful model in many US healthcare providers, such as the University of Pittsburgh Medical Centre, which is one of the largest healthcare providers in North America.

Private finance initiative

Many hospitals in England are actually owned by private companies under a PFI scheme. In this the company builds, services and owns the building for 30 or more years, while the NHS essentially buys the building and pays interest on the outstanding loan.

Independent sector

In the early years of the Labour government under Tony Blair, there was a desire to increase the capacity of the health services by introducing non-NHS providers from the independent sector. To remove the considerable barrier to entry for these new providers they were given contracts for volumes of clinical work by central government. Many built independent treatment centres which tended to focus on delivery of elective services.

Any willing provider

To create a competitive market, especially for elective services, the commissioners can invite in 'any willing provider'. All providers have to be accredited by the commissioner and licensed by the Care Quality Commission. However, on the approved list the provider can compete to offer services on the basis of a standard contract.

Novel joint structures

The Somerset Integrated COPD service is run by Bupa Home Healthcare in partnership with Avanaula Systems Ltd, a GP-owned business. They won the contract in competition with respiratory services from local hospitals and offer an at-home and community-based service with high levels of patient input.

General practices, polyclinics and poly-systems

These have traditionally been single-handed or owned by a partnership of GPs. There has been pressure to bring practices together to provide critical mass of a broad range of primary care staff. This may intensify with the increased regulatory burden of CQC licensing. Under the plan of Lord Darzi, Health Minister under Gordon Brown, larger entities termed polyclinics or, later, poly-systems were envisaged. In these, groups of practices brought together their resources and, with some transfer of funding from the hospital sector, were thought to be able to offer a broader range of services, with the intention of offering more care close to home and reducing the utilization of expensive secondary care.

Devolved administrations: Scotland, Wales and Northern Ireland

Scotland has 14 Health Boards covering the population and a number of non-geographical Boards such as NHS Quality Improvement Scotland, Scottish Ambulance Service, Scottish National Blood Transfusion Service, etc. The current Scottish Parliament is not seeking to introduce independent sector providers. The Boards have a close management relationship with the hospitals, GPs and walk-in centres.

Wales has also aimed to increase integration, with a reorganization in 2009 resulting in seven Health Boards and three NHS trusts (Welsh Ambulance Trust, Velindra Trust, which has a focus on cancer, and Public Health Wales).

Northern Ireland has an integrated health and social services system with four integrated Boards which monitor care delivered by local organizations.

Further reading

Feacham, R.A., Sekhri, N.K. and White, K.L. (2002). Getting more from their dollar: a comparison of the NHS with California's Kaiser Permanente. *British Medical Journal*, **324**: 135.

Chapter

34

Commissioning healthcare

There are two broad models of how a state-funded healthcare system can operate. Either the government gives each section a budget and the different parts of the service manage more or less well within the budget, or one part of the service acts as the taxpayers' agent and buys or commissions services from other parts which compete to offer the best service at lowest cost. This latter model mirrors the commercial world. This purchaser/provider split has been a feature of healthcare policy for nearly three decades. For the system to function, those who purchase or commission the service have to have a set of competences.

World Class Commissioning

The 2007 'World Class Commissioning' programme was an attempt both to define what commissioners have to do and to provide an assessment and national grading of how well they were achieving the task. The framework had a number of elements:

- Local leadership – the commissioners are supposed to be the leaders in the local NHS economy, enjoying a strong reputation with all the public sector organizations as well as the healthcare community
- Partnership working – the health of a community depends on local government, schools, housing policy, jobs, etc., and the commissioners have to work closely with those responsible for all issues which affect the health of a local population
- Engage the public – commissioners are buying on behalf of the public and need the public to buy into any plans
- Engage clinicians – commissioners need to have input from the whole clinical community in developing strategy and services and in ensuring quality
- Knowledge management – commissioning requires a great deal of knowledge in a very broad range of fields. The knowledge needs not only to be current but must anticipate changes in disease patterns and new technological advances. Prioritization decisions have to be evidence-based and there has to be an audit trail so that there can be challenges and appeals
- Needs assessment and prioritization – the commissioners need data and an in-depth understanding of the health needs of the community they serve. This should underpin their decision-making.
- Agents for change – commissioners should not be satisfied with the status quo but should stimulate the healthcare market, challenge existing providers and encourage new providers
- Drive for quality and innovation – the commissioners need to drive for continuous improvement by specifying quality and outcome targets they wish to see achieved on behalf of their population

- Procurement and contracting – commissioners need to be experts in the nationally regulated process of procurement and put in place proper contacts which protect the service and ensure value for money
- System management – commissioners manage the healthcare system and need to ensure via contract and outcome monitoring that the local population receives a sustained high quality service delivered by reliable resilient organizations
- Financial investments – commissioners are responsible for the money spent in the local healthcare economy. This will typically be many hundreds of millions of pounds. They are accountable for ensuring that the service is financially stable and that sound financial investments are made.

Commissioning going forward

The 2010 coalition government proposes to make major changes to the organization of commissioning, with GPs taking a lead role. There is also a proposal to move public health out of the commissioning team and place it in local authorities. Whatever the organizational structure and the re-allocation of roles between different bodies, it seems likely that most of the elements outlined in the World Class Commissioning programme will be required in some form or other.

Lessons from abroad

Many other countries have developed more sophisticated approaches to commissioning. These tend to rely on very well characterized datasets on patients. For example, in the USA the 'Pay for Performance' programme provides graduated payment to providers according to the percentage of patients with a particular problem who receive the complete care bundle or complete set of recommended discharge medication. Some commissioners analyse healthcare utilization by individual, and commission community intervention programmes to both monitor and provide a rapid response to those who have a track record of high utilization of secondary care.

Chapter

35

External regulators

QANGOs

Government has found it useful to have organizations a little distant from the central government departments to do some of its business. These are the quasi-autonomous non-governmental bodies (QANGOs), arm's-length bodies (ALBs), non-departmental public bodies and department-sponsored committees or organizations. The advantages are that they can have a constitution which encourages more public participation, they can bring well informed and often very gifted people from walks of life outside government to focus on an issue, and of course if there are problems they are easy to close down with little blame attaching to the minister. There are a large number in healthcare, and the number and structure is set to change under the policies set out by the coalition government.

Government organizations outside healthcare have regulatory roles, such as the Health and Safety Executive and the National Audit Office. In addition, there are a number of membership organizations that have regulatory functions, such as the GMC, and completely autonomous organizations which have contracts permitting them to comment or contribute to regulation.

The list below is not exhaustive, but tries to cover some of the main organizations or groups and gives a feel for the complexity of the regulatory framework in which healthcare is delivered:

NICE

The National Institute for Health and Clinical Excellence (NICE) is responsible for providing national guidance on promoting good health, preventing and treating disease. It produces (using a well established evidence-based methodology) a regular series of guidance for healthcare workers covering the full range of clinical areas. A very few have been very contentious. These have sought to limit access to expensive drugs on the grounds that the cost of the drug to the NHS does not justify the additional quality of life for the patient, measured as a QALY (Quality-Adjusted Life Years).

The Care Quality Commission

The Care Quality Commission (CQC) is the successor body to the Healthcare Commission and before that the Commission for Health Improvement. The CQC regulates care provided by the NHS, local authorities, private companies and voluntary organizations. From 1 October 2010, health and adult social care services in England have also required a licence. General practices and dentists are likely to be included in the requirement to have a licence. The idea is that all healthcare providers will require a licence, which is provided on the basis of achieving a set of standards. The licence can of course be revoked. The standards cover privacy and dignity of patients, hygiene and infection control, provision of basic care, patient safety, provision of adequately trained staff and quality monitoring.

NPSA

The National Patient Safety Agency (NPSA) has four main functions. It holds the national patient safety incident database, which is called the National Reporting and Learning System (NRLS). Every incident notified by a healthcare worker is copied to this database. From the database similar incidents are analysed and common causal factors are identified. The agency then works with service providers to provide generic solutions which are issued as safety alerts, and these are circulated to the service for implementation. As part of this the Agency runs the Patient Safety First campaign. The NPSA also has the National Clinical Advisory Service (NCAS), which advises organizations on how to manage a doctor who is exhibiting problems with conduct or competence. The NPSA has also recently had responsibility for the National Research Ethics Service.

The NHS Litigation Authority

The NHS Litigation Authority (NHSLA) handles all negligence claims against NHS organizations. These include clinical negligence and general claims – for example, for occupational injury. This area of work is similar to an insurance business and is funded by annual premiums from trusts. The NHSLA runs a scheme to improve risk management in trusts, which used to be called the Clinical Negligence Scheme for Trusts (CNST). Trusts are regularly assessed for both general services and maternity services. The higher the level of achievement in the assessment, the greater is the discount on the annual premium. The NHSLA is also responsible for resolving disputes between practitioners and primary care trusts, giving advice to the NHS on the Human Rights Act as well as handling some other areas of litigation involving the NHS.

Monitor

Monitor is the ALB responsible for regulating foundation trusts. Monitor is in close contact with the trust. Monitor checks performance against the annual plan and produces a regular risk rating on both governance (red, amber–red, amber–green or green) and finance (rated 1–5, where 1 is highest risk and 5 the lowest). If a foundation trust is at risk of breaching its terms of authorization, Monitor has the formal powers to intervene and ask for major management changes.

The Human Fertilisation and Embryology Authority

The Human Fertilisation and Embryology Authority regulates all fertility services, in particular in vitro fertilization, in the UK.

Health Technology Assessment

The Health Technology Assessment programme is part of the National Institute for Health Research and produces independent information on the effectiveness of new healthcare technologies.

The Human Tissue Authority

The Human Tissue Authority is responsible for licensing and inspecting organizations which store and use human tissue for research, treatment, post mortems, teaching, etc.

NHS Blood and Transplant Tissues Services

This organization collects, recovers, processes, banks and supplies blood and human tissues used as part of treatment within the NHS.

Foundation Trust Network

This is the organization that represents foundation trusts.

NHS Confederation

The confederation represents all NHS organizations and holds an annual meeting which is the major forum for communication of NHS business.

Medical Education England

Medical Education England (MEE) has a remit to coordinate training in medicine, dentistry, pharmacy and healthcare science.

Postgraduate Deanery

The Deanery has traditionally managed the process of postgraduate training, essentially buying training placements from hospitals, recruiting and monitoring trainees. This is likely to change, with the management of placements delegated to local commissioning based in selected large trusts.

General Medical Council

The GMC is a membership organization which is responsible for the registration and now licensing of medical practitioners. It has fitness to practise procedures to deal with those whose conduct or capability has been called into question.

National Confidential Enquiries

These are provided by independent companies. This independence means they can come to conclusions independent of input from government. They are also not subject to the same freedom of information requirements as government bodies. However, they rely on the voluntary reporting of events by frontline clinicians.

- NCEPOD – National Confidential Enquiry into Patient Outcome and Death
- CMACE – Centre for Maternal and Child Enquiries, including Confidential Enquiry into Maternal Deaths
- National Confidential Inquiry into Suicide and Homicide by people with mental illness (NCI/NCISH) is a research project run by Manchester University with funding from the public funds.

The criminal courts

Individuals can face criminal charges in respect of death of a patient. The organization can face charges of corporate manslaughter if there was a gross failure of management of health and safety leading to death.

Clinical Pathological Accreditation

Clinical Pathological Accreditation (CPA) is run by an independent company and provides a system by which pathology services can demonstrate by accreditation that they offer robust safe high quality services.

Royal Colleges and specialist societies

Royal Colleges and specialist societies are membership organizations which serve as the guardians of the knowledge base of medicine. They have a range of different remits for ensuring standards of training and developing improved ways of delivering services. They play a part in regulating by commenting on consultant job descriptions, participating in interview panels and inspections.

Organizations that ensure formal local community input

Over the past couple of decades a range of structures have been tried to ensure that there are formal structures for lay public input into healthcare. Community health councils were abolished and replaced by patient public forums. These have local involvement networks (LINks), with members working closely with individual trusts. Relations with local councils have been strengthened by ensuring accountability to the Overview and Scrutiny Committee. Coalition government plans may change the structure by the introduction of HealthWatch.

Ionizing Radiation (Medical Exposure) Regulations

Ionizing Radiation (Medical Exposure) Regulations require specific training and competence of all those involved in the use of ionizing radiation, and incidents have to be reported to and are investigated by the national lead.

Screening services

Breast cancer, cervical cancer, bowel cancer and, potentially, other cancers can be detected early by screening large populations within defined age bands. This is highly regulated. Adherence to protocols, proper use of resources and appropriate training are mandated. Any incidents are investigated in a prescribed way by the national leads.

NHS Business Services Authority

The Authority runs a number of businesses for the NHS. These include the pensions scheme, counter fraud, payment of pharmacists and dentists as well as playing a role in determining the price the NHS pays for consumables, especially medication.

Central Alerting System

The Central Alerting System brings together a range of safety alerts produced by the Department of Health, NPSA and MHRA. They are sent electronically to trusts and are available on a website. It is expected that NHS organizations will implement the recommendations of the alerts, and trusts are monitored against compliance.

Medicine and Healthcare products Regulatory Agency

The Medicine and Healthcare products Regulatory Agency (MHRA) is responsible for ensuring the safety of medicines and other products prior to their introduction into healthcare use in the UK.

Audit Commission

The Commission has played a role in the checking of value for money spent by public bodies. Some of its reports have related to the NHS. The coalition government have indicated that the Commission will be disbanded.

National Audit Office

The National Audit Office (NAO) audits public bodies, including money spent by the Department of Health. In 2010, The NAO produced a report indicating that the productivity of hospitals had fallen over the preceding decade.

Information Commissioner's Office

The Commissioner is responsible for ensuring openness by public bodies and also data privacy for individuals. The work covers the Freedom of Information Act in which public bodies are obliged to release information requested by a member of the public. The Commissioner has powers to fine organizations that lose personal data on individuals, such as hospital notes or any person-identifiable data.

Ombudsman

The Parliamentary and Health Service Ombudsman undertakes independent investigations into complaints that government departments and other public bodies have not acted upon properly and fairly. These reports are laid before parliament each year and attract press interest as well as potentially stimulating new regulation or legislation.

Coalition proposals

The landscape will change. The coalition government's review of regulatory bodies in July 2010 made the following recommendations regarding some of the above, and a number of other bodies:

- Alcohol Education and Research Council – abolish
- Appointments Commission – abolish
- Care Quality Commission – retain
- Council for Healthcare Regulatory Excellence (which oversees professional regulators) – make a self-funding body by charging a levy on regulators
- General Social Care Council (which regulates social workers) – transfer function to the Health Professions Council
- Health and Social Care Information Centre (which collects and provides health and social care information) – retain, focus on data collection with the NHS Commissioning Board

- Health Protection Agency (which protects the health and wellbeing of the population) – abolish and transfer functions to the new Public Health Service
- Human Fertilisation and Embryology Authority – retain as a separate ALB for the time being
- Human Tissue Authority – retain for the time being
- Medicines and Healthcare products Regulatory Agency – retain
- Monitor – retain and make an economic regulator, operating a joint licensing regime with CQC
- National Institute for Health and Clinical Excellence– retain
- National Patient Safety Agency – abolish as an ALB. Safety functions transferred to the National Commissioning Board. Explore transfer of National Research and Ethics Service functions to single research regulator. National Clinical Assessment Service to become self-funding over the next 2–3 years
- National Treatment Agency for Substance Misuse (which works to increase the availability, capacity and effectiveness of drug treatment in England) – abolish and transfer functions to the new Public Health Service
- NHS Blood and Transplant – retain, and make more commercially effective
- NHS Business Services Authority – retain in short term
- NHS Institute for Innovation and Improvement (which supports the NHS by spreading new ways of working, new technology and leadership) – remove from ALB sector
- NHS Litigation Authority – retain and explore greater commercial involvement.

Chapter

36

Treatment centres

Since the early 1990s, clinicians in the NHS have been advocating the separation of elective from emergency surgical care, in order to improve productivity and relieve pressure on the acute sector. Day surgery units were developed as early models of elective surgery centres. In 1999 the first treatment centre in England dedicated to a wider range of elective procedures was opened at the Central Middlesex Hospital. In 2002, the Department of Health announced that it was creating a programme of similar NHS treatment centres, including a number of independent sector treatment centres (ISTC).

The aims of the Treatment Centre Programme were to:

- Provide the extra clinical capacity needed to deliver swift access to treatment for NHS patients
- Spearhead diversity and choice in clinical services for NHS patients
- Stimulate innovative models of service delivery
- Drive up productivity.

Treatment centres are now well established in the UK. These centres concentrate on the efficient delivery of high volume elective diagnostics and surgical procedures. They vary in the types of services they offer and focus on reducing waiting times in locations and specialties with particularly large numbers of patients on waiting lists. From 2005, NHS patients have had a choice of up to five providers when needing hospital treatment and many have taken up offers of swifter treatment in one of these centres.

How are they funded and where are they sited?

Treatment centres are funded through NHS public capital, private finance initiatives, independent sector money or a combination of these, including public–private partnerships. Many are stand-alone new builds while others are situated on refurbished sites or in mobile units. They are purpose designed to maximize efficiency and streamline patient flows.

What are their benefits?

The creation of these centres has meant that patients:

- Wait less time for routine operations
- Have a choice about where and when they are treated
- Are looked after by specialist teams
- Do not have their operations cancelled for non-clinical reasons
- Are treated in comfortable, modern surroundings.

In addition, acute hospitals benefit as pressure on beds is relieved, speeding up treatment for emergency patients. Staff work on a planned patient list each day and so their working hours are largely predictable. For workers with family responsibilities this can be particularly valuable.

How are they staffed?

Treatment centres are staffed in a number of ways:

- Entirely by NHS staff
- A mix of NHS and independent sector staff
- A mix of NHS and overseas staff
- Entirely by independent sector staff.

The staff who work in the NHS centres are employed in exactly the same way as other NHS employees, while those in ISTCs will normally work under independent sector terms and conditions. In some instances, NHS staff may also work in ISTCs under structured arrangements and retain all the benefits of NHS employment terms and pension rights.

How are they regulated?

There is a fundamental requirement for treatment centres to have in place formal govern-ance procedures and quality assurance systems. They are monitored in the same way as any other NHS hospital.

Independent sector treatment centres

ISTC services are provided by the private sector. The centres were set up to provide additional capacity. Many of the ISTCs are stand-alone sites, physically removed from local acute hospitals. They are managed by independent healthcare organizations from across the world. The Department of Health premise was that contracts for services were to be secured under a competitive tendering process and based on value for money. The first wave contracts included a stipulation of 'additionality' and financial guarantees, whereby ISTCs were assured of a certain level of income irrespective of how many procedures they performed for the NHS. The initial contracts were for 5 years and they were prohibited from employing anyone who had worked for the NHS in the previous 6 months. Partly as a result of this, ISTCs were overwhelmingly staffed by overseas clinicians.

The ISTC contracts are funded from local primary care trust (PCT) budgets and the services delivered are part of the overall requirements of local delivery plans. As the ISTCs are delivering NHS services, free at the point of delivery and available according to clinical need, they carry NHS branding. Patients have the same rights as they do in any other NHS hospital or healthcare facility. All surgeons working in these centres have to be registered with the GMC and be on its specialist register. All centres are monitored for clinical outcomes, hygiene and patient satisfaction. They are also subject to NHS peer reviews by local clinicians and are expected to have in place quality assurance and quality improvement systems.

The House of Commons Health Committee review of first wave ISTCs concluded that these had not made a major direct contribution to increasing capacity and that they were not necessarily more efficient than NHS treatment centres. They also could not find convincing evidence that techniques pioneered in the ISTCs were being adopted in any systematic way in the NHS. A number of concerns were raised about the ISTC programme by the professional medical bodies and others. There were concerns that ISTCs were poorly integrated into the NHS and that they were not training doctors. Concerns were raised about clinical quality and continuity of care. There was also considerable scepticism about whether the ISTC programme represented value for money. The Department of Health had failed to assess and quantify fully the effect of competition and destabilization on local NHS services.

In 2005 the Department announced the commissioning of a second wave of ISTCs and promised to address some of the anxieties that Phase 1 had created: additionality would be restricted to increase the involvement of NHS staff and improve integration; all ISTCs would offer training and secondments to NHS staff.

Key points

- The 'challenge' of ISTCs may have galvanized improved efficiency in the NHS. However, there have been other drivers for efficiency, namely additional NHS spending and waiting list targets
- ISTCs may cherry-pick cases, taking the simpler and more profitable cases, leaving the more complex ones to the NHS
- If complications occur in an ISTC, the patient may need to be transferred to an NHS hospital and the NHS then needs to pick up the tab for dealing with the complication
- There are worries about the vetting and appointment procedures for European Economic Area qualified doctors
- There is no convincing evidence that ISTCs provide better value for money than NHS treatment centres or partnership arrangements
- Contracts between PCTs and ISTCs contain guaranteed levels of income for the ISTCs. As a result there is a powerful incentive to PCTs to encourage patients to use ISTCs rather than NHS treatment centres
- There are real concerns that the expansion of the ISTC programme will destabilize local NHS trusts, especially those with financial difficulties.

Further reading

General information about treatment centres. www.dh.gov.uk/en/Healthcare/Primarycare/ Treatmentcentres (accessed 5 April 2010).

House of Commons Health Committee Report. (2006). Independent sector treatment centres. www.publications.parliament.uk (accessed 5 April 2010).

37

Who does what – the trust Board

What does the Board do?

The Board is the tap that controls resource allocation. The Board directly, or via delegation according to the predefined delegation of authority, controls all spending in the organization. The Board:

- Formulates strategy in line with the demands of the external environment
- Allocates money via the annual budget or via business case approval in line with the strategy
- Holds the organization to account, via the Executive team, to ensure the money spent delivers the pre-agreed volume of activity and quality and to ensure no overspend against budget. Holds the Executive to account for ensuring the organization follows the strategy and delivers change to the agreed timetable. The Board holds the accountability for the organization in the eyes of the external world
- Shapes the culture of the organization.

Delegated authority levels: the Board delegates authority to spend money. All NHS organizations will have a delegated authority policy which indicates the levels of expenditure allowed by each post in the organization. If an order for a higher amount is needed, the individual has to obtain sign-off from a more senior member of staff with a higher delegated level.

Core structure

Boards in the NHS have a reasonably standard structure:

- The chair and non-executives must be equal or greater in number than the Executives
- Must include as a minimum the chief executive, finance director, medical director and nurse director, commonly also the chief operating officer
- May include non-voting directors, e.g. estates, HR, IT, director of corporate affairs, etc.
- Certain Boards have specific additional requirements; for example, most teaching hospital trusts have a university representative as a non-executive.

Governance structure

The governance structure can vary but needs to answer the following challenges.

- How does the Board know what is happening in the organization?
- How does the Board assure itself that the organization is performing well?
- How does the Board know that the organization is as good as or better than other similar organizations?

- Where is the paper trail of evidence in the event of a catastrophe and external inquiry to protect Board members and show that they had been monitoring the organization?

There has been a growing emphasis in all organizations on Board accountability and governance following scandals such as Enron, and reports by Cadbury, Greenbury, Hampel and Higgs. NHS Boards are no exception. Indeed, the fact that NHS organizations are spending taxpayers' money voted by parliament to be used for the purpose of helping the sick and preventing disease imposes a greater burden on the NHS for good governance and open accountability. Decisions need to be taken by those with the proper authorities, according to predetermined protocols and with records made by the appropriate committees. The outcomes of decisions need to be monitored. External overview and scrutiny is essential. Risks need to be identified and managed. The recent inquiry by Robert Francis QC into quality failing at the Mid Staffordshire foundation trust has further raised the accountability of the Board for the quality of clinical care.

Audit Committee

The Audit Committee is a statutory subcommittee of the Board. It will be chaired by a non-executive director who is not the Board chair. The committee challenges the Executive to ensure that money has been spent on the purposes intended, and that it has delivered best value. The Audit Committee is fed data and analysis by internal audit and by the external auditors.

Internal audit

The finance department employs or buys services from a small team of individuals who conduct internal audits. The annual audit plan is agreed at the beginning of the year on a number of days per task basis. Internal audits usually have a strong financial element and focus on demonstrating good use of resources. Typical topics might include adherence to best practice in procurement, or closer to the medical staff, attendance by consultants at direct clinical care sessions on their job plan.

External audit

At the end of the financial year all the income and expenditure of the organization is checked by an external firm of accountants. This process culminates in a management letter from the accountants and determines whether the annual accounts can be issued without any qualifications. In practice there is substantial dialogue through the year. The external auditors are interested in ensuring that the organization offers best value for money and will be involved in a number of studies comparing financial spend in different areas of the organization with the performance of other similar organizations.

Annual accounts

All commercial bodies are obliged to produce annual accounts. The annual accounts comprise a text section about the performance of the organization and a detailed financial section. These are public documents. They are presented once a year to an annual general meeting or to the annual meeting of the members in the case of foundation trusts.

Quality accounts

This new requirement attempts to match financial accountability with a rigorous accountability for quality.

Risk management

This is an essential function of the Board. The Board has to review Serious Untoward Incidents, aggregate data on clinical incidents, complaints, health and safety issues (in particular radiation accidents) and occupational injuries such as sharps injuries. The Board reviews the Risk Register, which collates all risks identified and stratified on the basis or severity and likelihood of recurrence.

The Board also has to review the Board or Trust Assurance Framework, which is subtly different. The Assurance Framework attempts to look forward and asks what might stop the organization doing what it wants to do. The Assurance Framework thus provides the trust with a method to monitor the risks to meeting its strategic objectives. It also enables the Statement of Internal Control, which in turn shows that the management has got control over the business now and is going forward.

The Risk Committee is another subcommittee of the Board, usually chaired by a non-executive director who is not the chair of the Board, charged with ensuring that things which might go wrong have been identified and that all reasonable steps to mitigate the risks have been taken.

All NHS bodies are required to prepare public statements to confirm that they have done their reasonable best to maintain a sound system of internal control to manage and achieve their objectives. This is achieved by the chief executive providing a signed statement of internal control which is usually supported by the Trust Assurance Framework.

Clinical Governance Committee

All trusts have a Clinical Governance Committee which reports directly to the Board or via the Audit or Risk Committee. Different trusts have different structures to their Clinical Governance Committee. Whatever the structure, there are a number of common functions:

- Provide assurance to the Board on the clinical quality
- Interrogate and hold to account departments and teams
- Provide an outlet for problems
- Ensure that actions to improve quality are implemented
- Monitor quality and key performance indicators
- Ensure patient safety compliance
- Drive better clinical performance.

Remuneration Committee

The pay of the chief executive and those who report directly to the chief executive is determined by the Remuneration Committee. The pay, including any pension entitlements of executive and non-executive directors, is made public in the annual accounts. Very senior managers, defined as those who report to the chief executive, are exempt from 'Agenda for Change'. There is Department of Health guidance on 'Very Senior Managers' pay issued by NHS Employers.

In some categories of NHS organization the Remuneration Committee can award bonuses on the basis of performance when the individual and organization have achieved or exceeded the annual objectives. Traditionally there is a relationship between reward in terms of pay and risk, and in terms of liability to loss of job owing to poor performance. There is also a recognized link between pay and the leverage an individual has over the performance of the organization. There have been many examples of rapid departure of a chief executive, more commonly because of patient safety problems than financial failure.

External Board accountability

The chief executive is the accountable officer to parliament for the spending of public money. In practice, that accountability is through the strategic health authority. In a foundation trust the Board is accountable to the governors and through them to the wider membership. This arrangement attempts to mimic corporate shareholders in the commercial world, since there are usually over 10 000 members from all parts of the local community, including staff, who have a clear vested interest in the success of the trust.

Board personality

All Boards comprise people. Since the Board is the most senior part of the organization, the people on Boards tend to be ambitious, driven and interested in power and control. The personalities of the key people have a major impact on the personality of the organization and on how people within the organization behave. If the chair or chief executive is a bully, then senior managers may also resort to bullying. If the Board is led by people with a particular interest, that will be reflected in investment decisions and in the interest of the whole organization. Spending time and some resource on Board development is essential, to ensure that this group of key people work together and that their overall contribution is greater than the sum of the parts.

The Board cycle

The management consultant and academic Bob Garratt has argued that the Board functions fit naturally into an annual cycle. This naturally matches many of the functions of an NHS Board:

- Strategy review looking outside the organization to position the organization in the changing market. Sign contracts and budgets
- Operations review, with performance management to ensure delivery
- Governance review to ensure organizational compliance
- Policy review to create a culture and ensure the internal parts of the organization support the strategy.

Chapter 38

Who does what – the Executive *et al.*

The core functions of the Executive team are planning and control. The questions posed by the team are: What does the external world need us to do for the business to thrive? What risks have we got to deal with? Do we have a plan? Are we in control of the organization or is it freewheeling out of control?

Executive structure

The core members of the Executive are the chief executive, the finance director, the medical director and the nurse director. In most trusts there is also a chief operating officer, a director of human resources, a director of estates and often a director of IT. There is a regular Executive Committee meeting which allocates resources and monitors performance. Allocation of resources has to be achieved with the proper audit trail to show how the decision was made, and this starts with a business case that is submitted for approval. Performance monitoring addresses the full range of the organization's functions and asks was performance delivered and was value for money achieved?

Role of the medical director

In most trusts the medical director is responsible for some or all of clinical quality and patient safety, and directly or indirectly for all matters relating to the medical workforce. He or she may cover any number of the other responsibilities which fall to the Executive, such as infection control, complaints and in some organizations a substantial proportion of the operation's function, communications or strategy development. The medical director is not the doctors' lobbyist on the Board. However, he or she will need to ensure that the Executive and Board are well advised on clinical best practice and that there is a good relationship between management and the medical staff.

Clinical/medical management structure

Most hospitals have a clinical division or clinical directorate structure. Traditionally these have been on professional lines with, for example, separate directorates for medicine and surgery. Some trusts have experimented with a more functional structure, separating emergency and elective care into separate directorates. There are inherent advantages and disadvantages in any structure. For example, it is easier to manage individuals of the same specialty together; however, having surgeons and anaesthetists in separate parts of the organization can cause tension when trying to organize operating schedules.

Clinical directorates are led by a medical member of staff who works closely with a senior manager and senior nurse. The relationships between these individuals and an appropriate balance of power within this triumvirate are essential to success.

In most trusts there is some form of divisional representation on the trust Clinical Governance Committee. The growing emphasis on accountability will probably change this arrangement and require the clinical director to be able to give the Executive much greater assurance of the quality of care in his or her directorate.

Typical medical director reports

Staff who work in the following areas commonly report to the medical director: medical education, research and development, some elements of patient safety, clinical risk management, medicolegal and clinical governance. The HR issues of appraisal and performance management are more commonly in HR but may move with revalidation and the creation of the Responsible Officer role.

Education structure

There is usually a trust Education Board with a subcommittee for medical education. The medical education function is often so substantial as to justify at least one member of the consultant body leading on medical education and reporting to the medical director.

Typical internal expert advisory committees

In a hospital there are many areas that need monitoring and improving where the professional expertise of the clinical staff is essential. Most hospitals have a number of committees to focus on areas such as medicines management, drugs and therapeutics, blood usage and venous thromboembolism prevention. These are professionally led and report to one of the statutory subcommittees of the Board such as Clinical Governance.

Typical time-limited working groups

There are multiple tasks that the organization has to address which commonly require a short-term committee to meet regularly and deliver a piece of work. A classic example might be a cost improvement programme committee, with a task to reduce the expenditure of the organization.

Direct reports to other members of the Executive team

There are a range of activities and teams that report to different members of the Executive team. Most are obvious, with all of finance, payroll and internal audit reporting to the finance director and all the operations staff reporting to the director of operations. Typically, complaints and patient experience report to the nurse director. Infection control has to be led by a director of infection prevention and control (DIPC) who has to report directly to the chief executive. The DIPC may be the nurse director or someone outside the Executive team, in which case infection control staff will report to another Executive.

Operations management

The core task of operations management in any organization is to balance three variables: cost of production, the volume of production and the quality of the product. In hospital terms this equates to balancing costs, the level of activity or patient flow, which in turn often relates to how fast patients are seen, and the quality of care or the safety of patients. Change any one of the three and there will likely be an impact on at least one of the other two. The challenge is to optimize all three.

Line management

Everyone in the organization reports to a 'boss'. That person in turn has a line manager. Each management line ends with one of the executive directors. They in turn report to the chief executive. This accountability is exerted both through the line of authority and budgetary control. It is important that these two lines run through the same individuals.

Who is the consultant's boss?

The chief executive is the ultimate boss of all consultants. In the UK most consultants report to a clinical lead who in turn reports to a clinical director. In most trusts the clinical director reports directly to the chief operating officer or chief executive, since this is also the budgetary line. In some trusts the clinical director may report directly to the medical director, and the budgetary line runs through the general managers to the director of operations. In the USA the medical management line is often very separate from the management line organizing the nurses and other aspects of care. In this situation the two lines have to negotiate to create joint working. This can pose difficulties in team-working, and in the UK there is greater emphasis on managing clinical service teams as one, irrespective of the professional makeup of the team.

Chapter

39

Activity and targets

Setting a target is a way for the government to ensure that the vast NHS focuses on a priority and achieves something that the government can then use to identify to the voter and taxpayer what their money is achieving.

The 1997–2010 Labour government markedly increased funding for the NHS and introduced a number of targets. Examples of 2009 targets follow.

Acute hospital service standard targets

Number of A&E attendees waiting less than 4 hours	>98%
Patients with cancelled operations receiving operation within 28 days	>95%
MRSA bacteraemia cases above hospital-specific target	'x'
Clostridium difficile patients above hospital-specific target	'x'
Patients waiting less than 18 weeks from GP referral to start of treatment	>90%
Patients contacting genitourinary medicine (GUM) clinic to be seen within 48 hours	>98%

Cancer targets

There were multiple targets for patients with suspected cancer, requiring less than 2 weeks for GP referral to attendance at the relevant clinic, treatment to be commenced within 62 days, and any second or subsequent treatment within 31 days.

Impact of targets

Within each of these targets there were a very specific set of definitions specifying exactly which patients and which situations were within and outside the scope of the target. The existence of targets changed behaviour and a large proportion of hospitals in England achieved all or some of the targets. For example, in 1997 waiting over 18 months for elective surgery on the NHS was common, but by 2010 waiting over 18 weeks was a rarity. Not all of the clinical community were happy working in what some perceived as a target-driven world.

The coalition government have said that they wish to move away from top-down targets and have national outcome standards. They anticipate having relatively few targets and to ensure that these have an evidence base supported by NICE. Given that the government is accountable for taxpayers' money, it seems unlikely that there will be no national standards against which to measure service performance.

Irrespective of the national requirements, the local commissioners have the flexibility to include targets in their annual contract. Hitherto these have largely followed the government standards.

Clinical process redesign and lean thinking

Delivery of healthcare is achieved by a multitude of interconnecting processes, delivered by a changing population of staff and using a vast range of ever-evolving technologies. The system of integrating these into the clinical process must develop and change.

The value chain

What is the value chain? Typically, organizations focus on the activities they undertake on behalf of the customer. Analysis of the value chain asks what benefits the customer receives from these activities. For example, a hospital is often focused on whether to invest in the latest diagnostics equipment which may help to refine a diagnosis in a relatively small number of cases, but is probably available at a neighbouring hospital. However, a dominant concern from patient groups is the problem with finding spaces in the hospital car park.

Lean pathway design

Lean pathway design examines in detail the process for a specific clinical pathway, listing every step and every interaction. Those steps that add value are identified, those required by regulation are identified and those steps that create no value but merely generate activity are eliminated. Commonly the remaining steps in the pathway need to be re-ordered.

Where the ideas came from – Deming and Toyota

W. Edwards Deming, an American academic, developed the concept of statistical process control. He was frustrated his ideas were rejected in the USA and he moved to Japan where he worked with Toyota. His concept was to simplify the production process, introduce 'just in time' thinking and total quality management. Statistical methods were used to study production quality. If we think outside medicine, it is easy to see the benefit of such an approach. If all the ball-bearings used in an engine are exactly the same size, it is likely that the engine will break down less frequently than if there were to be 2% variation in the diameter of the ball-bearings. The question is how to bring this level of rigour to healthcare delivery.

The mathematics of process design

We might think that achieving success with $P > 0.95$ is pretty good. However, in a pathway of 10 steps, the cumulative chance that all steps will occur correctly is 0.95^{10} or 0.6 or 60%.

The more steps, the worse the chance that all will occur correctly. Even if each step occurred correctly 99 times out of 100, a pathway of 100 steps would happen in an error-free way less than 40% of the time.

The solution is to reduce the number of independent steps and to make downstream steps dependent on the success of the critical upstream steps. This reduces the length of independent sequences of steps. In effect it also allows the pathway to be able to check its own performance.

Steps in lean process redesign

- Map the whole process from beginning to end – write each step on a sticky note and stick the notes in order on a board. Include all the steps, including correspondence, phone calls and patient/notes/sample movement between departments as well as patient movement to and from home
- Identify improvement opportunities – evaluate steps for how they add value to patient care. Rearrange the notes
- Smooth the flow – smooth the journey and remove the barriers to the smooth even flow of patients
- Create 'Pull'– organize so that later stages pull patients through the earlier steps. For example, in an emergency pathway create a system where the general medical wards and the specialist physicians are driving to get patients out of A&E onto their wards rather than the A&E staff trying to push patients onto the general wards
- Hold a 'rapid improvement' event – in this, staff come together to make a step change. For example, machines may need to be moved or clinical areas reorganized to support the new way of working
- Continuous improvement – staff need continually to revisit the pathways and continuously improve.

Key issues

- It should feel better – simpler better managed pathways result in less unnecessary work, fewer mistakes, better patient safety and cost reduction
- All staff from consultants to porters must participate
- Commonly, areas of activity of low value are identified and the feelings of staff have to be protected
- A facilitator and patient input may be helpful.

Removing waste

Seven types of waste have been described and should be eliminated:

- Injuries – damage to people, stress and start injury patients
- Defects – stuff that is not right and needs to be fixed, e.g. clinical complications
- Inventory – stuff waiting to be worked on, e.g. patients on waiting lists
- Over-production – too much stuff, e.g. unnecessary tests or X-rays
- Waiting – people waiting for staff to arrive, e.g. patients waiting for a ward round before discharge
- Motion – unnecessary human movement, walking up and down
- Transportation – moving stuff or patients.

Lean pathways and skill-mix

What categories of staff should best undertake each of the steps? What is the optimal mix of skills required? From a cost-efficiency perspective, it is desirable that the most expensive staff (usually senior doctors) undertake only those steps for which they are uniquely qualified. This principle can be pushed all the way down the clinical team.

Examples of lean approaches in healthcare

Care bundles

There is considerable evidence that, whilst clinicians know the five or six things which need to be achieved for a particular condition, in practice most patients receive only a subset of the required interventions. Care bundles are a system of grouping all the required interventions and ensuring that all of them are completed on every patient. There is considerable evidence now from the USA and the UK that this approach saves lives and cuts costs.

'Just in time'

Why store resources, why not get them 'just in time' for when you need them? This is cheaper since storage and holding stock costs money and this makes work flow simpler. But the process has to be very well organized.

Six Sigma

We would very rarely expect an event to occur more than three standard deviations from the mean. Six Sigma is a technique where the events in the production process are measured and there is a focus to ensure that all occur within three standard deviations on either side of the mean.

Theory of constraints

This theory forces an examination of the bottlenecks to a process. If the bottlenecks cannot be removed or bypassed, then the speed through the slowest step in the process will determine the rate of flow of the whole process and this needs to be factored into operations planning.

Walk-in walk-out hernia service

Traditionally when a patient presented with a hernia, there were a series of letters, appointments, tests, pre-admission assessment, admission procedures, etc. In a walk-in hernia service, the GP books the patient straight onto the day case local anaesthetic list. The patient attends and leaves after surgery an hour or so later.

One-stop shop

Similarly, services for cervical nodes or breast symptoms can be organized so that all necessary diagnostic procedures are provided in the one visit.

Show and go

The conventional model in an imaging department is for the patient to arrive with a request form and receive an appointment to return for a test at a later time or date. Since across a year all those who attend with a request form receive the test, why do we insert a delay and require the patient to wait. In a 'show and go' service, when the patient shows up, they get the test and then go.

'Walk-in' GUM

Prior to the government target that all patients attending a genitourinary medicine (GUM) clinic had to be seen in 48 hours, a typical clinic gave appointments and patients sat for long periods in a waiting room waiting. The target forced a radical change. Now patients are seen on presentation. Some clinics have reorganized to open from 7am to 7pm and monitor time spent by the patient on the premises to keep near to 30 minutes.

Pre-op assessment

The introduction of generic pre-op assessment clinics run by nurses with support from anaesthetics has streamlined pre-op processes and reduced the number of patients attending for an operation who are unfit for surgery.

Enhanced recovery programme

In the enhanced recovery programme, pre-op patient education, modifications of the anaesthetic protocols, use of minimally invasive surgery, altered post-op pain control and mobilization have allowed marked reductions in length of stay. Some patients are able to have less than a 24-hour stay for a colon resection and have a 1-day length of stay for a hip replacement.

New to follow-up ratios

Once a diagnosis is established and the first step of treatment is arranged, why do we follow patients up in the hospital clinic? If provided with an appropriate clinical algorithm, the patient and the GP between them are usually perfectly capable of ensuring satisfactory chronic disease management for most common conditions.

Patient empowerment – copying letters to patients, patient information and education

The patient lives day to day with their disease. The more they understand about it and the management plan, the greater their potential contribution to ensuring satisfactory disease management. Information transfer is essential via copying letters to patients, providing written information and individual or group education of patients. For example, in maternity, women attend antenatal classes, have a birth plan and hold their own notes, but this is poorly developed in other areas of healthcare.

Smaller waiting areas

If you walk through a large clinic such as a fracture clinic you will see very many people waiting. Often the number waiting exceeds the number of chairs and there is a proposal to expand the waiting area and increase the seating. In lean thinking, the answer is that keeping patients waiting adds no value to the patient or service. In fact, the size of the waiting area should be decreased and the flow of patients through the clinical area should be increased via use of more clinical staff, more efficient patient flows or reducing the requirements for follow up.

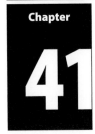

Chapter

41

Managing change

Managing the status quo is hard enough – how can you manage change?

There are many web documents and a multitude of people who make a living helping teams through the process. The core principles are to engage everyone, use evidence, make a plan, implement the plan and monitor the outcome. It sounds easy but is in fact very difficult. Below are a number of elements which are useful.

Organizational approaches

Seven S

Originally devised in 1980 this provides seven dimensions against which to examine an organization – structure, strategy, systems, staff, skills, style of management and shared beliefs (or culture). Successful organizations have these seven elements organized in such a way that they are mutually supportive. For example, if the business systems and structure are very rigid and hierarchical but the culture is relaxed and style of management casual, the organization is unlikely to work well. Ask the following questions: what are we trying to do, what is our strategy? What skills do we need for this (both clinical and managerial), what types of staff do we need and with what training? What organizational structure will deliver change and what organizational systems will support what we want to do? What style of management and what culture will ensure that the change is implemented? What stories, heroes, rewards and celebrations will back up what we want to do?

PESTLE

The organization needs to look at its business environment to work out what to do and develop a strategy. The teams need to consider external issues under a number of headings: political (P), economic (E), sociological (S), technological (T), legal or regulatory (L) and environmental (E). For example, what is the impact of new government policy or a new diagnostic screening test going to be on my service?

SWOT

Given the external environment, what are the strengths (S), weaknesses (W), opportunities (O) and threats (T) facing my service?

Stakeholder mapping

Who outside and inside the organization will benefit or be disadvantaged by any change we make? These are the stakeholders. Make a list of all of them. For each person or group, what is their level of commitment or compliance with what you might want to do? What is their readiness and their capability to give support and help? People might want to help but have no time or money. A small minority who will be disadvantaged can bring any project to a halt, however sensible the original idea appeared to be. So these people need to be won over from the start.

Force field analysis

The status quo exists because the forces driving change are in equilibrium with the forces restraining change. When attempting to create change it is preferable to reduce the restraining forces because this allows movement, without increasing tension. Group norms are an important force in resisting and shaping organizational change. This technique requires listening to people; understanding the impact of established work patterns, complacency and possible job insecurity on people; and then thinking of creative ways to re-align restraining forces.

Learning organization

The underpinning principle is that the ability to learn faster than competitors may be the only sustainable competitive advantage. The organization needs to institutionalize learning how to do things better and to regard continual change as the norm. The corollary is that working in an unchanging way should make you nervous that somehow you are getting behind. The focus is on systems and their interrelationships. An example might be that rapid patient flow through A&E requires all parts of the emergency pathway from the front desk of A&E, to the final dispensing of take-home medication for long-stay admissions, to be continuously reviewed and improved.

Context, content and process model

The approach considers change in three dimensions. There is a context, both external (see PESTLE above) and internal (including internal resources, capabilities, culture and internal politics). On the content axis, there is what the project entails, such as the objectives, assumptions, targets, milestones and evaluation. On the process axis there are the approaches to change, such as who will do it using what model and with what plan.

Problem-analysing approaches
Fishbone diagram

In analysing a problem it soon becomes apparent that the main problem has many contributory factors and these in turn have further contributory factors. The fishbone diagram tries to illustrate these on one piece of paper. The main problem has a timeline which is the backbone of the fish going from left to right across the page. At different times along this timeline major contributory factors play a part represented by diagonal lines going up or down like fish bones and intersecting the main backbone. Similarly, along each of these diagonals, smaller lines intersect, showing how the second generation of contributory factors interact.

Five whys

This approach is useful for looking at one problem event. Interrogate the cause by asking the question 'why?' at least five times. For example, suppose there is a clinical incident where a deteriorating patient was not seen quickly. The first 'why' might show that the junior doctor did not attend for an hour. Why? – Because he or she was at a teaching session.

Why? – Because his or her teaching had been scheduled to clash with ward duties. Why? – Because the schedule was out of date. Why? – Because the person who wrote the schedule was on maternity leave and the task had not been reallocated.

Operational approaches
Total quality management (TQM)
Most industries have given a great focus to improving the process of production of whatever their product is. TQM identifies 10 core principles to help with this.

- Productive work is achieved via processes. In these every worker does part of the process. In so doing, they supply to the next person in the chain for them to do their part of the process, and receive from, or are a customer of, the person in the preceding part of the chain. There are thus within the process of production a multitude of customer/supplier relationships which have the ability to go wrong
- These relationships need to be measured, clarified and improved
- Most quality defects are due to process not individuals
- Preventing defects is cheaper than detecting them later
- Understanding variability of processes is key to increasing quality. Quantitative measurement of outcomes and reduction in variability of outcomes is key
- Quality control should focus on the 'vital few' processes not the 'useful many'
- Measurement is essential, e.g. what the customer needs and what the customer receives, as well as process stability and variability
- Total employee involvement is critical
- New structures such as a Quality Council may help
- Integrate quality planning, quality control and quality improvement. Thus define the level of quality you want to achieve, measure outcomes and continuously improve.

Control charts
These charts have time on the horizontal axis and the relevant quality measure on the vertical axis. In any day or week there will be subtle variation in quality. The chart can be analysed by producing a regression line to show trend of improvement and by drawing confidence intervals indicating the lines three standard deviations from the mean. Values outside these confidence or control lines need investigating since they are unlikely to have occurred by chance and suggest a problem with the business process.

Business process re-engineering
The premise is that business processes need to be re-thought and radically redesigned to achieve dramatic improvements in cost, quality, service and speed. The concepts are that organizations should be organized around process rather than specialist functions; that narrow specialists should be replaced by multi-skilled workers often working in self-managed teams; that radical re-thinking and change is needed rather than incremental improvement espoused by TQM; that this must come from top management and that intensive hands-on management is needed. A possible example might be a day case operating facility where surgeons, anaesthetists, theatre staff and recovery staff all work as one team and to some extent share roles.

Focus on the value chain

This asks you to identify and focus on the value chain (see Lean thinking).

Gantt chart

A Gantt chart is like a spreadsheet with each column comprising a regular time interval, e.g. month 1, month 2, etc. Each row corresponds to a task which needs to be completed. The chart documents the start and end of the task, with a solid line between these points identifying when the task will be in progress. This layout allows tasks to be planned and re-ordered in accordance with their dependency relationships so that tasks that have to come first are scheduled first. Also, it allows resources to be deployed in a sensible way so that later tasks actually are undertaken later. The chart also serves as a monitoring tool so that, as time goes by, it becomes clear if all the tasks are being completed by their anticipated date and, if not, the consequences for later tasks can be identified.

Motivating staff

Mission statement

Most organizations have a short pithy statement that focuses everyone's mind on what the job actually is. This allows people to ask themselves whether what they are doing is in line with the mission statement. If it is not then they need to question whether they should re-focus their energies. For example, Salford Royal NHS foundation trust has a statement 'We aim to provide safe, clean, and personal care to every patient, every time.'

Organizational values

If the organization has clearly articulated values that everyone shares, this will support change if it is in harmony with the values. Most NHS organizations have a fairly broad set of published values covering patient care, quality, safety, respect and excellence. In some trusts, departments have developed very focused value statements. It is often the process of defining the values with all the members of the team that brings the department together. As an example, one of the values of the cardiology department at the Royal Berkshire foundation trust is: 'We have a commitment and passion for what we do, and believe that this is reflected in the service we deliver and the disposition of our staff.'

Appreciative enquiry

The principle is to build on what works, rather than focus on the negative. A substantial number of staff in the organization contribute to creating a list of what about their work makes them feel good. Groups are asked to talk about a good day at work, what they did and why it went well. From this, the values that support this good work are distilled and reinforced across the organization.

Change cycle (PDSA)

The NHS Institute have espoused a cycle of change with four stages. Plan (P), in which the change is planned; do (D), in which the change is tested or performed; study (S), in which the effects of the change are studied; and act (A), in which the change is fully implemented or the next change cycle is planned.

Staff engagement

Classic behaviours and attitudes have been identified which make change difficult. These are hopelessness, cynicism, distancing and blaming others. These are the symptoms of organizational malaise. They need to be addressed by engaging staff with the management agenda, sharing the management problems and taking ownership by the staff of the problems. There is an argument that the frontline staff are the only people who know the solutions. It is just that no one member of the frontline staff has all the solution, only one small part. So the job of management is to collect the elements of the solution from the members of staff and assemble it.

Critical success factors

These are things you must have to succeed. In a change programme, critical success factors might include internal leadership of change; clinical ownership and support for change; weak resistance to change; external support for change both politically and materially; partnerships of clinicians and managers leading the change; objectives of change that incorporate professional development, service development or service problem-solving; formal and informal communications processes.

Further reading

http://www.sdo.nihr.ac.uk/files/adhoc/change-
    management-developing-skills.pdf (accessed
    27 December 2010).

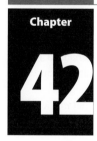

Patient safety

Patient safety is one of the most important aspects in healthcare delivery. This has been emphasized with the publication of the government White Paper 'Equity and Excellence: Liberating the NHS' in July 2010, which puts increased safety at the heart of its proposals.

Improving patient safety involves assessing how patients may be harmed, preventing or managing risks, reporting and analysing incidents, learning from such incidents and implementing solutions to minimize the likelihood of them happening again.

There are no definitive figures available for adverse events relating to patient safety, but various estimates are available. In 2000, the Department of Health (DoH) published 'An Organization with a Memory', the report of an expert group on learning from adverse events in the NHS. This report suggested that every year:

- 400 people died or were seriously injured in adverse events involving medical devices
- Nearly 28 000 written complaints are made about aspects of clinical treatment in hospitals
- The NHS pays out around £400 million each year in settlement of clinical negligence claims, and has a potential liability of around £2.4 billion for existing and expected claims
- Hospital-acquired infections are estimated to cost the NHS nearly £1 billion.

Other research-based estimates suggest that in NHS hospitals adverse events in which harm is caused to patients occur in around 10% of admissions. Although serious failures are uncommon, when they do occur they are often caused by weak systems rather than the fault of any one individual. In addition, and of equal importance, some specific types of relatively rare but very serious adverse events happen repeatedly.

Key reports

Several key reports have been published in relation to patient safety. These include:

- An Organization with a Memory (2000)
- National Audit Office Report: A Safer Place for Patients – learning to improve patient safety
- Safety First: a report for patients, clinicians and healthcare managers. Published in December 2006. It was commissioned by the Chief Medical Officer to reconsider organizational arrangements in place to ensure that patient safety is at the heart of the healthcare agenda
- Health Select Committee Inquiry into Patient Safety. The House of Commons Health Select Committee (HSC) published its report on patient safety on 3 July 2009. The government response to the HSC report was published on 13 October 2009.

The National Patient Safety Agency

The National Patient Safety Agency (NPSA) opened in 2001 and is a Department of Health arm's-length body (ALB); these are stand-alone national organizations sponsored by the DoH that work closely with hospitals, social services and other ALBs. They are accountable to and receive substantial funding from the DoH.

In the past few years the NPSA has led the drive to improved, safe patient care by informing, supporting and influencing organizations and people working in the health sector. It is comprised of three divisions with separate roles and responsibilities.

National Reporting and Learning Service

The National Reporting and Learning Service (NRLS), established in 2003, manages a national reporting system on behalf of the NHS in England and Wales. The system enables patient safety incident reports to be submitted to a national database and this information is analysed to identify hazards, risks and opportunities to improve the safety of patient care.

From 1 April 2010 it became mandatory for NHS trusts in England to report all serious patient safety incidents to the Care Quality Commission as part of the Care Quality Commission registration process.

Other services provided by the NRLS include:

- The production of safety alerts related to a wide variety of topics
- The 'seven steps series'.

The seven steps series provide a checklist to help clinical staff optimize all aspects of patient safety. They all provide guidance so that when things do go wrong the right action is taken. They also help trusts maintain clinical governance commitments. The steps are:

- Build a safety culture
- Lead and support your staff
- Integrate your risk management activity
- Promote reporting
- Involve and communicate with patients and the public
- Learn and share safety lessons
- Implement solutions to prevent harm.

There are four 'seven steps' guides available: these are for general patient care, primary care, general practice and mental health.

National Clinical Assessment Service

The National Clinical Assessment Service (NCAS) was formed in 2001 to help in situations where there is concern about a doctor's, dentist's or pharmacist's performance. It offers advice, specialist interventions and shared learning. It aims in its guiding principles to be effective, authoritative, objective and fair.

National Research Ethics Service

The National Research Ethics Service (NRES) has two goals for research in the NHS. The first is to protect research participants who take part in clinical trials and other research within the NHS. The second is to promote ethical research that is of potential benefit to participants, science and society. NRES aims to fulfil these roles in various ways, including:

- Supporting research ethics committees (RECs)
- Providing a quality assurance framework for the research ethics service
- Providing a training programme
- Promoting transparency in research.

Future of the NPSA

The DoH report of 2010, 'Equity and Excellence: Liberating the NHS', set out plans for reform of the NHS. This publication contained details of plans to reduce the numbers of ALBs, including the NPSA, from 18 to 10. The safety function of the NPSA will be retained and transferred to the National Commissioning Board. The function of the NRES at the NPSA is likely to be transferred to a single research regulator, and the NCAS is expected to become self-funding in the next 2 years.

Never Events

Never Events are serious, largely preventable, patient safety incidents that should not occur if the available preventative measures have been implemented. Primary care trusts are required to monitor the occurrence of Never Events within the services they commission and publicly report them on an annual basis. The Never Events Annual Report 2009/10 provides an overview of the Never Events reported to the NPSA by NHS organizations in England from 1 April 2009 to 31 March 2010.

An engagement exercise on the future of Never Events for 2011 and beyond for the NHS is being led by the Department of Health. Further information is available on the Department of Health website http://neverevents.dh.gov.uk (accessed 6 January 2010).

The core list of Never Events:

- Wrong site surgery
- Retained instrument post-operation
- Wrong route administration of chemotherapy
- Misplaced nasogastric or orogastric tube not detected prior to use
- Inpatient suicide using non-collapsible rails
- Escape from within the secure perimeter of medium or high security mental health services by patients who are transferred prisoners
- In-hospital maternal death from post-partum haemorrhage after elective Caesarean section
- Intravenous administration of mis-selected concentrated potassium chloride.

Further reading

http://www.npsa.nhs.uk/ (accessed 6 January 2010).

http://www.nrls.npsa.nhs.uk/neverevents/ (accessed 6 January 2010).

Chapter

43

Recent disasters in healthcare in England

Harold Macmillan, the British prime minister from 1957 to 1963, when asked about obstacles to political achievement, said 'Events, dear boy, events'. Events have been a major change agent for British healthcare over the past couple of decades. A number of scandals have led to a public outcry for greater regulation of healthcare delivery. This section provides brief details of some of the more high profile disasters.

Wayne Jowett

Wayne Jowett was 18 and in remission with leukaemia when he died at the Queen's Medical Centre in Nottingham in 2001 after intravenous vincristine was wrongly administered via the intrathecal route. The responsible doctor, Dr Mulhem, who was only 3 days into his first post as a specialist registrar in haematology, had instructed a junior doctor to inject an anticancer drug into the patient's spine. Within a few minutes the doctor realized the magnitude of his mistake. After pleading guilty to the manslaughter of his patient by gross negligence, Feda Mulhem was given a custodial sentence of 8 months.

This case and the report 'An Organization with a Memory' led to the creation of the National Patient Safety Agency (NPSA).

Bristol babies

Between 1988 and 1995, at the Bristol Royal Infirmary, the cardiothoracic surgeon Mr Dhasmana carried out 38 arterial switch operations in which 20 of the children died. Between 1990 and 1994, his colleague Mr Wisheart carried out 15 atrioventricular septal defect operations. Nine of the children died.

These two surgeons at Bristol Royal Infirmary, Mr James Wisheart and Mr Janardan Dhasmana, and the former chief executive Dr John Roylance were found guilty of serious professional misconduct by the GMC, Mr Wisheart and Mr Dhasmana for continuing to operate on infants when the death rate was unacceptably high, and Dr Roylance for not intervening.

A Public Inquiry by Sir Ian Kennedy produced close to 200 recommendations. These included the following.

- Children – children in hospital must be cared for in a child-centred environment, by staff trained in caring for children and in facilities appropriate to their needs
- Safety – the NHS must root out unsafe practices. It must remove barriers to safe care. In particular, it must promote openness and the preparedness to acknowledge errors and to learn lessons. Healthcare professionals should have a duty of candour to patients
- The competence of healthcare professionals – it must be part of all healthcare professionals' contracts with a trust (and part of a GP's terms of service) that they

undergo appraisal, continuing professional development and revalidation to ensure that all healthcare professionals remain competent to do their job

- Organization – all employees should be treated in a broadly similar manner. Doctors, nurses and managers must work together as healthcare professionals, with comparable terms of employment and clear lines of accountability, in order to provide the best possible care for patients
- Standards of care – there must be agreed and published standards of clinical care for healthcare professionals to follow, so that patients and the public know what to expect. There must also be standards for hospitals as a whole. Hospitals that do not meet these standards should not be able to offer services within the NHS
- Openness – there must be openness about clinical performance. Patients should be able to gain access to information about the relative performance of a hospital, or a particular service or consultant unit
- Monitoring – there must be effective systems within hospitals to ensure that clinical performance is monitored. There must also be a system of independent external surveillance to review patterns of performance over time and to identify good and failing performance.

These recommendations have been central to the change in accountability for clinical work in UK hospitals over the past decade. They have led to internal hospital regulation and enhanced national regulation and scrutiny.

Rodney Ledwood

Rodney Ledwood was struck off the medical register in September 1998 after a review of 150 operations showed that a third had complications which were probably due to negligence. There was great concern that it had taken 15 years for his incompetence to come to light, prompting calls for greater outcome monitoring.

Harold Shipman

In 2003 a 54-year-old GP from Hyde, Greater Manchester, Harold Shipman, was jailed for life for the murder of 15 of his patients. He subsequently committed suicide in jail. An inquiry identified up to 250 patients who potentially died at the hands of Dr Shipman. After an extensive inquiry and detailed report, the last part of which was published in 2005, there were recommendations for major changes to the monitoring of medical practitioners. The report has led to the introduction of revalidation and forced a re-organization of the GMC.

Kerr and Haslam

William Kerr and Michael Haslam were convicted in 2000 and 2003, respectively, of indecent assault at the same psychiatric hospital in North Yorkshire where they worked during the 1970s and 1980s. The victims were vulnerable female psychiatric patients who had gone to their consultants for treatment. The question raised was how the behaviour of the two doctors went unquestioned for so long. The investigation took the view that many colleagues were kind and caring, there was no deliberate conspiracy to cover up sexual misdemeanours but rather that warning bells were ignored or dismissed and some people remained silent when they should have spoken out.

Alder Hey inquiry

This inquiry, published in 2001, investigated the removal, retention and disposal of human organs and tissues following post-mortem examinations at the Royal Liverpool Children's Hospital NHS trust between 1988 and 1995. In many cases, these organs were removed without informed consent, were not subsequently subjected to histological examination nor used for educational or research purposes, and preliminary post-mortem reports were left unfinished. The investigation identified failures within the hospital, the university and the Coroner's Office, which had allowed the systematic removal of organs. This inquiry led to the Human Tissue Act, requiring consent to be obtained for the retention of post-mortem material and clear documentation and regulated storage.

Bedford bodies in the chapel

In 2001 it came to light that dead bodies had routinely been stored in the hospital chapel during busy periods over the preceding 5 years. The chief executive, Ken Williams, resigned. This incident reinforced the importance of ensuring that the deceased were treated with dignity and respect by hospitals.

Stoke Mandeville *C. difficile* outbreak

Between October 2003 and June 2004 Stoke Mandeville Hospital had 174 cases of *Clostridium difficile* infection and in a second outbreak between October 2004 and June 2005 a further 160 cases. Of the 38 patients who died in the outbreaks, 33 definitely contracted the infection after being admitted to the hospital. The Healthcare Commission found that 41 patients had probably died from the organism and it had contributed in a further 24 patients. The managers were criticized for prioritizing political targets, such as reducing waiting times, over patient safety. During the first outbreak at Stoke Mandeville senior managers ignored calls by doctors and nurses to isolate infected patients in order to meet the government's target for a maximum waiting time in A&E of 4 hours. This led to patients with diarrhoea being kept in or put on open wards. During the second outbreak managers decided to close an isolation ward against the advice of both the hospital infection control team and the Health Protection Agency (HPA).

This report came at a time when there was a 17.2% increase in cases of *C. difficile* in hospitals throughout England, with over 50 000 cases in 2005.

Maidstone and Tunbridge Wells *C. difficile* outbreak

There was a similar outbreak of *C. difficile* at Maidstone and Tunbridge Wells Hospital, investigated in 2007 after there had been up to 90 deaths. The trust was heavily criticized about cleanliness, hygiene and infection control.

These outbreaks led to a major set of initiatives by the government to reduce hospital-acquired infection. Despite initial cynicism from the medical profession, the reduction in *C. difficile* and MRSA infection in hospitals has been dramatic. The latest data from the HPA website suggest that *C. difficile* infections in the over-65 age group in UK hospitals fell from over 8500 in the quarter from April to June 2008 to under 5500 in the quarter from April to June 2009.

Basildon

The Care Quality Commission performed an unannounced inspection in October 2009 to assess the risk of healthcare-associated infection at Basildon and Thurrock University Hospitals NHS foundation trust. They found areas of concern and issued a warning notice. This was followed up by another unannounced inspection on 5 December 2009. Poor nursing and a dirty clinical environment were identified and heavily criticized. It is believed that this may have contributed to a higher than average A&E mortality rate.

Mid Staffs

The inquiry into the Mid Staffordshire NHS foundation trust was triggered by a persistent increased hospital risk-adjusted mortality rate, particularly for emergency patients. Examples of appalling care and a failure to prioritize the care of the patient over achievement of targets and financial surplus have been heavily criticized. For example, patients were left in soiled bed linen and relatives took sheets home to wash. Since the trust was a foundation trust and enjoyed a degree of 'hands off' supervision from the local NHS, the scandal has raised questions about the governance arrangements for foundation trusts. The implications of this scandal may yet continue and affect the freedoms offered to foundation trusts and the type of regulation and monitoring to which they are subject.

Conclusion

The period of the Labour government in the UK from 1997 to 2010 coincided with a large number of high profile scandals in healthcare. This led to a loss of confidence in professional self-regulation and pressure on the government to introduce external monitoring processes on medical staff and healthcare delivery in general.

Further reading

http://www.dh.gov.uk/prod_consum_dh/ groups/dh_digitalassets/@dh/@en/ documents/digitalasset/dh_4065086.pdf (accessed 27 December 2010).

http://www.bristol-inquiry.org.uk/final_report/ Summary.pdf (accessed 27 December 2010).

Safety and quality

Litigation

When a medical error occurs and a patient is harmed, the patient or the bereaved will be looking for an explanation, an apology and reassurance that the same thing will not happen to someone else. They may also be looking for financial compensation to recompense them for loss sustained as a result of the error and sometimes as a means to obtain retribution. Different countries deal with this in different ways according to their legal systems. In the UK the issue of harm caused by negligence is covered by civil law. Negligence is a tort: an act or omission that causes harm to an individual's property, reputation or interests. The law of tort imposes a duty of care where one party could reasonably foresee that his or her conduct may cause harm to another. In most cases of medical negligence, the claimant has to prove that he or she has suffered injury or other harm because of the negligence of the healthcare provider. Some medically negligent conduct may also constitute a criminal offence.

To support them in the event that this occurs, all doctors are required to have medicolegal insurance cover. When a GP is sued he or she is defended and insured by his or her defence association – usually the Medical Defence Union or the Medical Protection Society. The situation is similar for private practice. For allegations of negligence in hospitals, the NHS organization carries the indemnity and is effectively insured by the government via the NHS Litigation Authority (NHSLA), which was formed in 1995.

At the time of writing the NHSLA is a special health authority with the primary roles of managing clinical and other liability claims made against NHS organizations in England and promoting good risk management. The NHSLA also monitors human rights case law on behalf of the NHS, runs the Family Health Services Appeals Unit (which resolves disputes between primary care trusts, GPs and others who provide primary care services) and advises on management of equal pay claims in the NHS. The NHSLA functions in a similar way to an insurance company, and each scheme is a mutual pool, funded on a pay-as-you-go basis, by annual contributions from its members.

The fact that within the NHS it is the clinicians' employers, usually NHS trusts, rather than the individuals themselves, that are deemed to hold the duty of care to patients is of vital importance. If the employer carries the liability then the employer has considerable power over what the employee is allowed to do.

Large sums of money are involved. The NHSLA spends around £1.3bn per year on claims and makes an accrual in its books of £13bn in relation to future claims. The annual income to pay for the claims comes mainly from the trust in the form of an annual premium referred to as CNST payment (Clinical Negligence Scheme for Trusts). The value of the premium varies according to a number of factors but is counted in numbers of millions of pounds. The NHSLA receives some Department of Health funds for its other functions.

There are five key issues in medical negligence:

- **Was there negligence?** An early precedent was provided by the Bolam proceedings of 1950. The case provided the so-called Bolam test, which provides a defence if the individual has acted 'in accordance with practice accepted as proper by a responsible body of medical opinion'. The strength of the Bolam test has been eroded over the past 20 years. There is much greater reliance on evidence-based medicine, published data and compliance with the large number of national and specialty-based guidelines. A central part of defending any case is good contemporaneous documentation.

- **What is the quantum of loss?** The loss sustained by the plaintiff has to be expressed in cash terms. There is often considerable argument over the extent that injuries have actually translated into financial loss or additional living expenses, which comprise the compensation claimed.

- **How will the lawyers' fees be paid and by which party?** Traditionally the losing side pays all the fees. The recent introduction of 'no win no fee' arrangements by plaintiff solicitors and the practice of advertising to potential victims has changed the pattern and cost of claims. Plaintiff lawyer costs have risen markedly. The fees for winning a case are allowed to be high to compensate for those cases lost. However, the solicitors presumably recruit a large number of potential cases and become very competent at only accepting those where there is a strong chance of winning.

- **Over what time period will the payment be made, as a lump sum or annually over the lifetime of the patient?** These latter periodical payments have the advantage of ensuring, particularly for high value birth injury cases, that money continues to be available to provide care in the long term. However, there has been debate over the index used to increase the value of the annual payment to compensate for inflation. A recent judgment gave permission for this to be calculated using indices reflecting inflation in care workers' salaries. It is feared that over time this index may turn out to be higher than the retail price index and cause cost inflation.

- **How is a balance struck when trying to resolve litigation?** At least as far as the NHSLA is concerned, there are two difficult balances to be struck when trying to resolve litigation. At a strategic level the government has a duty to defend its employees and conserve taxpayers' money, but it also has a duty to ensure the citizen is protected, has easy access to justice and is compensated for any properly assessed losses due to negligence which might otherwise fall to other aspects of the welfare and social services budgets for the state to support. The second balance is struck on a case by case level when the cost of fighting a case which might or might not succeed has to be balanced against the cost of settling a case quickly and cheaply. There have been cases where a consultant has been upset that a case has been settled where he has felt he was in the right but where the commercial decision was to settle the claim and make a relatively small immediate payment when taking into account the possibility of losing and the large additional costs which would then be incurred.

Other ways of resolving medical negligence

There has been some discussion on creating an NHS redress scheme in which at least small value cases are settled by some sort of panel without recourse to the courts, following a model developed in New Zealand. This has not progressed in the UK since the plaintiff would always have the right to go to court if he or she was not satisfied with the outcome.

What is the advice on offering an apology?

The NHSLA, the defence societies and the BMA have agreed a position statement on what to do and say if something goes wrong. This is available on the NHSLA website. All parties recognize that the facts will come out during any legal process and it is better to investigate the incident locally and be honest with the facts. The statement encourages you to give apologies along the lines of 'I am really sorry that this set of circumstances happened'. The statement makes the point that, as the involved clinician, you are too close to events and are not in a position to make a judgement over negligence. This needs the objectivity of others outside the clinical situation and needs to take into account wider information on case law. Similarly, you as a clinician are not in a position to make any comment on the quantum of any loss.

What to do if a claim arrives?

When a letter of claim arrives, immediately discuss it with the relevant legal services team in the hospital or, if you are a GP or the incident occurred in private practice, with your defence society. The legal team will manage the process. You will be invited to review the notes and make a detailed statement. You may subsequently be invited to put together evidence from the literature or guidelines to support what you did. If the case is likely to go to court, you may also at a later stage be invited to a case conference with a solicitor or barrister to discuss the details. If the case is going to court you should be offered and would be well advised to accept some training in presenting your case in a courtroom setting. In some cases, an adverse outcome of a court case will precipitate a referral to the GMC. Involvement in a legal case is often associated with considerable fear, guilt and anxiety, and can cause great stress and upset. Good advice is to stay calm, talk to the legal team and your clinical or medical director.

What is likely to happen to the claim?

Around 40% of claims are ultimately dropped, 40% are settled out of court, 15% take a very long time to resolve and around 5% are settled in court. The highest value cases are birth injury cases and these are the ones which take longest to resolve.

Preventing claims

The best protection is to have well thought through policies and procedures which make sure the organization is well run, that high quality staff are employed and appropriately trained, and that in every clinical situation staff follow best practice every time and keep appropriate records. This is easier to say than to achieve. To encourage best behaviour the NHSLA have created a set of risk management standards for general trust services and for maternity services. Trusts are assessed regularly against these standards. Achievement of the standards at higher levels attracts a discount on the annual CNST premium.

Safety and quality

Clinical governance

Clinical governance is a system for maintaining and improving the quality of patient care within the health system. It is defined as 'a framework through which NHS organizations are accountable for continually improving the quality of their services and safeguarding high standards of care by creating an environment in which excellence in clinical care will flourish'. This definition embodies the concepts of high care standards, transparent accountability and improvement. As the name implies, clinical governance relates to the delivery of care to patients and their carers but this is also interlinked to the organization of healthcare services. The term 'integrated governance' is used to refer jointly to corporate governance and clinical governance within healthcare organizations.

The legal responsibility for clinical governance lies with the trust Board of each hospital, with the chief executive of the trust ultimately the person who is accountable. Although the chief executive and the trust Board are responsible, they cannot do all the work by themselves. Their role is therefore to make sure that there are structures in place to ensure that clinical governance is fully embedded at all levels. Practical responsibility for clinical governance is delegated to the medical director, nursing director, clinical directors and consultants. Ultimately everyone in the hospital is responsible for ensuring that standards of care are constantly maintained and improved. Each trust must prepare an annual quality report, summarizing the quality of care delivered and the implementation of good clinical governance.

The elements of governance
There are at least seven elements of governance.

Education, training and professional development
The individual and the trust have a responsibility to ensure that all staff are up to date and maintaining continuous professional education and development. In practice, for doctors this involves attending courses and conferences, indulging in self-directed lifelong learning, taking relevant exams, workplace-based assessments and appraisals.

Clinical audit
Clinical practice must be reviewed and the performance measured against agreed standards. This process must be cyclical, and regular re-audit of practice should occur to ensure that safety and clinical effectiveness are maintained. The overall objective of audit is to improve clinical care and outcomes and this is encouraged throughout all stages of a doctor's career.

Clinical effectiveness and research

Clinical effectiveness means ensuring that everything you do is designed to provide the best outcomes for patients. All doctors must perform and re-evaluate the clinical effectiveness of the treatments and interventions that they perform. The difficulty with this relates to whether a particular intervention is appropriate and whether it represents value for money. This is possible by adopting an evidence-based approach in the management of patients, developing new guidelines and protocols, implementing NICE guidelines, National Service Frameworks and other national standards to ensure optimal care.

Research helps to develop the body of evidence that establishes best practice. Clinical practice must change in respect to emerging new evidence from research. All doctors must carry out critical appraisal of relevant literature and implement research evidence into their clinical practice.

Openness, patient and public involvement

The needs of a trust's catchment population should be sought, understood and catered for. This means that there must also be openness between the local authorities and any health communities as well as the trust and the representatives of the community that the trust serves. Patient and public involvement is important in the development of services and the monitoring of treatment outcomes. This is possible through national patient surveys, local feedback questionnaires, patient advice and liaison services (PALS), local public networks (LINks) and through appointment of lay members to boards and committees.

Quality assurance must be maintained through appropriate internal systems and external regulation. This ensures that any problems with poor practice or performance are not managed in a 'closed door' environment. All systems and processes, whilst protecting the patient and supporting the practitioner, must be open to public scrutiny.

Risk management

Risk management involves having robust systems in place to understand, monitor and minimize the risks to patients and staff, and to learn from mistakes and near misses. It includes complying with protocols, policies and procedures, critical incident reporting and promoting a blame-free culture to encourage reporting of problems and errors.

Staffing and staff management

This relates to the need for appropriate recruitment and management of staff, ensuring that under-performance is identified and addressed, encouraging staff retention by motivating and developing staff and providing good working conditions. Safety and quality are key priorities for the NHS, with safety being considered as an 'absence of unacceptable risk to a patient'. All trusts must employ high quality employment practices and a safe environment for patients and practitioners.

Using information and information technology

This relates to the need to ensure that patient data is held securely, patient confidentiality is respected, patient data is accurate and up to date and data is used to measure outcomes and to develop services.

Clinical governance by doctors cannot be successfully implemented without the support of the non-clinical aspects of healthcare delivery. The support of administration and clerical staff, human resources, finance and information technology needs to be utilized to ensure that effective clinical governance is undertaken by doctors.

Further reading

NHS Confederation. www.nhsconfed.org (accessed 4 December 2010).

Scally, G. and Donaldson, L.J. (1998). Clinical governance and the drive for quality improvement in the new NHS in England. *British Medical Journal*, **317**: 61–5.

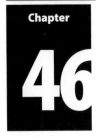

Risk management

Incidents

'If you do not know about it, you can't fix it' is a philosophy espoused by the Veteran Administration Healthcare System in the USA. Every NHS institution has an incident recording system. This requires the incident to be graded and prompt relevant local investigation to be carried out. If serious, a more formal internal investigation must be undertaken by the organization.

Serious untoward incidents

A serious untoward incident (SUI) is a category of serious incident for which a specified procedure must be followed, including reporting to external authorities and the Board of the trust. An SUI requires investigation in more depth. The criteria which trigger an SUI include unanticipated death or serious harm, following a clear failure of what is regarded as a normal service, especially if the incident is likely to attract media attention or cause public concern.

Root cause analysis

Root cause analysis (RCA) is an approach to investigation which drills down to all the causes and contributory factors that caused the incident. This starts with a timeline of all the events and brings in contributory factors which in turn may have their own timelines. Techniques such as fishbone diagrams and the five whys may be used. Collecting written statements from staff as near to the time of the incident as possible is essential.

NPSA decision tree

In deciding the extent to which it is appropriate to allocate blame to any individual it is important to have completed the investigation and to understand the precise contribution of the individual to the incident. The NPSA has a decision tree on the website to help. If the person was doing their best in good faith but lacked training, or had been placed in a situation where they were out of their depth, then support and training are likely to be needed. If the person was ill, or under the influence of drugs or alcohol, then a different approach is needed. In extreme cases, where a person was reckless and ignored the advice of others or deliberately set out to cause harm, a procedure to address failings in conduct or capability would be likely to be more appropriate.

Implementation of actions to improve safety

An understanding of the causes of an incident should prompt an action plan to prevent future incidents. At a later date it is also important to have an audit to ensure implementation of the actions has been sustained.

Risk register

The risk register provides a way for the organization to ascertain what might go wrong. The register lists all the issues that might go wrong. The risks are identified by a top-down and bottom-up process. Thus the Executive identify corporate risks and each ward, clinical team or division identify risks, and these are all collated. The risks are all scored. Each risk is scored from 1 to 5 on the basis of the qualitative magnitude of the severity. The risk is also scored from 1 to 5 on the basis of the likelihood of a recurrence. The scores for each risk are multiplied together to give a combined score with a maximum of 25. Risks are ranked in the register by combined score. Risks with a score of greater than 15 are regarded as high or extreme (Table 46.1). The process can be difficult and is subject to value judgements, but there is a guidance template to help assess the magnitude of the severity. Risks can change rapidly and the process has to be repeated regularly.

The Risk Committee meets regularly (approximately every quarter) and requires the Executive to have taken actions to reduce the likelihood and severity of the risks, starting with those that have the highest score. Commonly this requires expenditure which, according to the amount, may require Board approval. An example of a high risk might be the discovery that there is *Legionella* in the water supply. A clinical example for many trusts in 2009 was the consequence affecting both financial and clinical risk of the introduction of the European Working Time Directive. Another example of extreme clinical risk might be a number of incidents where individuals had received the wrong dose of radiotherapy.

Incidents and complaints

Incidents and complaints are an important feed into the risk register. Aggregated themes which underpin multiple incidents and complaints constitute by definition risks which recur and cause harm to patients.

Health and safety

Health and safety is a statutory responsibility. All trusts will have a Health and Safety Committee and/or designated office. The committee will report directly or indirectly to the Risk Committee since health and safety risks will be prominent on the risk register.

Facilities and environment issues

There are a number of safety issues such as the fire safety certificate, water quality and *Legionella* testing that relate to the physical plant of the hospital, which, if deficient, have a high priority on the risk register.

Table 46.1 Qualitative risk assessment matrix

(Likelihood × Severity = Level of risk)						
		LIKELIHOOD ⟶				
		Unlikely 1	Low 2	Moderate 3	High 4	Certain 5
SEVERITY	1 No harm or near miss	1	2	3	4	5
	2 Minor	2	4	6	8	10
	3 Moderate	3	6	9	12	15
	4 Major	4	8	12	16	20
	5 Catastrophic	5	10	15	20	25
Level of risk						
		No or low risk (green)	Moderate risk (yellow)	Significant risk (orange)	High/extreme risk (red)	
		1–3	4–6	8–12	15–25	

Corporate Manslaughter Act

The Act introduced the offence for organizations of gross failures in the management of health and safety with fatal consequences. An organization is guilty of the offence if the way in which its activities are organized by its senior management amount to a gross breach of the duty of care it owes to its employees, the public or other individuals, and those failings caused the person's death. This act emphasized the importance for hospitals of using the risk register to actively seek out things that could go wrong and having a realistic and well managed plan to reduce the chance of an incident or accident causing a fatal event.

Summary

The risk register is a 'safety net' for all. There are those who sometimes feel that services are unsafe. The way to bring these concerns into focus is via the risk register. Inevitably management has to prioritize where to invest. This investment decision-making will be informed by the risk register. If a doctor feels there are concerns, he or she needs to notify incidents, participate in investigations and ensure that relevant concerns are fed into the risk register. These will be scored and those conferring the greatest risk will be first in line for investment. This allows medical staff to discharge their responsibility to raise concerns and allows management to demonstrate that they have responded.

Chapter

47

Ensuring quality

The NHS is committed to providing high quality care. Quality and safety criteria are set and monitored nationally, with every organization's performance assessed and made public.

'The New NHS: Modern, Dependable', the Labour government's first health policy White Paper (published in 1997), promised that the service 'will have quality at its heart'. Eleven years later and coinciding with the 60th anniversary of the NHS in July 2008, the Next Stage Review's final report 'High Quality Care for All' defined quality from a patient's perspective as comprising: patient safety, patient experience and effectiveness of care.

NHS organizations have a statutory duty to ensure the quality of their services. Under the Health Act 2009, all providers of NHS care have to publish 'quality accounts' indicating the quality of care they provide. Other recent measures designed to foster quality include Commissioning for Quality and Innovation (CQUIN), adjustments to the tariff system to link increases in payments to specific quality goals and registration with the Care Quality Commission.

As commissioners, primary care trusts (PCTs) are held to account for the quality of health outcomes they achieve for their populations, including the most vulnerable and those with complex needs. A 'quality observatory' to enable services to be benchmarked is also being set up by each strategic health authority.

Quality accounts

Quality accounts must include the following:

- A statement of accountability from the provider
- Priorities for improvement and reporting arrangements to track progress
- A review of quality performance, confirming that the organization has set indicators for patient safety, effectiveness of care and patient experience, is developing a quality improvement plan and participates in clinical audit
- Confirmation that the organization uses CQUIN
- Reports on what others say about the provider, such as reports from the Care Quality Commission.

Commissioning for Quality and Innovation

The CQUIN payment framework makes part of a provider's income conditional on quality and innovation. It allows PCTs to link a specific proportion of the provider's contract income to locally agreed quality goals. All CQUIN schemes will be required to include a patient experience element. From 2011/12 on, PCTs will be able to withhold a significant proportion of contract payments if providers fail to meet agreed patient satisfaction goals for every service they provide.

Quality and Outcomes Framework

The Quality and Outcomes Framework (QOF) is an incentive scheme to encourage high quality services in general practice. This was introduced in 2004 and sets out a range of national standards based on the best available research evidence. The standards are divided into four domains:

- Clinical standards linked to the care of patients suffering from chronic disease
- Organizational standards relating to records and information, communicating with patients, education and training, medicines management and clinical and practice management
- Additional services, covering cervical screening, child health surveillance, maternity services and contraceptive services
- Patient experience, including assessing access to GP appointments measured by the GP patient survey.

A set of indicators that are reviewed annually by NICE has been developed for each domain to describe different aspects of performance. Practices are free to choose the domains they want to focus on and receive payments against the indicators, which are adjusted according to list size. About 15% of practice payments nationally are made through QOF.

NICE quality standards

NICE is developing a library of 150 quality standards, derived from the best available evidence from NICE guidance or other sources accredited by NHS Evidence. Produced in collaboration with health and social care professionals, they will help to end variations in care quality.

Indicators for Quality Improvement

Working with professionals right across the NHS, the NHS Information Centre and the Department of Health have identified an initial, but evolving, set of indicators to describe the quality of a broad range of services – the Indicators for Quality Improvement (IQI). These 200 or so indicators cover the three dimensions of quality: safety, effectiveness and patient experience. They are primarily intended for use by NHS staff to inform quality improvement activities, and are supported by appropriate statistical techniques to analyse and interpret the data. (www.ic.nhs.uk/mqi, accessed 28 December 2010.)

National Service Frameworks

National Service Frameworks (NSF) or 'National Clinical Strategies' are evidence-based programmes setting quality standards and specifying services that should be available for a particular condition or care group across the whole NHS. They are intended to eradicate local variations in standards and services, promote collaboration between organizations and contribute to improving public health. NSF strategies exist for:

- Paediatric intensive care
- Mental health
- Hypertension
- Chronic obstructive pulmonary disease
- Coronary heart disease

- Cancer
- Older people
- Diabetes
- Renal services
- Children, young people and maternity services
- Long-term conditions.

Care Quality Commission

The CQC was set up in 2009. Its role is to regulate health and adult social care services. Since 2010, health and adult social care providers must register with the CQC to provide services. The CQC assesses providers against core standards, national priorities, financial management and their use of the Mental Health Act and the Mental Capacity Act. If organizations fail to meet the regulatory requirements, the CQC can levy fines, impose conditions on registration, suspend registration or prosecute for certain offences. The coalition government is committed to strengthening the CQC's role.

National Quality Board

An initiative of the Next Stage Review, the National Quality Board provides strategic oversight and leadership in quality across the service. It is chaired by the NHS chief executive and includes the following members: the NHS medical director, chief medical and nursing officers, chairs of the CQC, NICE and Monitor, leaders from charity sectors, academia, social care and the Royal Colleges.

The Board's role is to 'align quality at all levels in the NHS'. It oversees work to improve quality indicators, advises the Secretary of State on priorities for clinical standards set by NICE and reports annually on the state of quality using internationally agreed measures.

Further reading

Care Quality Commission. www.cqc.org.uk
(accessed 28 December 2010).

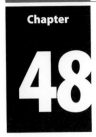

Chapter

Quality indicators

Assurance and quality

It is vital that any organization can give assurance to the owners (in the case of the NHS, the government and the voters), the users or patients, and the staff, that the quality of care is high. The Francis report following the exposure of poor quality care at the Mid Staffordshire Hospital Trust resulted in every member of every Board of any NHS organization being reminded of his or her personal responsibility for quality. This created a step change. Where previously people might have been happy to hear a report of 'no problems', now the organization is required recurrently to prove that quality is good. The challenge is to determine what we can measure to do this. This area of 'Ward to Board assurance' is a dynamic one and the list of topics is evolving.

No one number captures the whole picture. It is important to measure a number of different parameters and to ensure both internal and external perspectives are included. Wherever possible, data needs to be benchmarked and trended over time. The measures need to look at the inputs to the clinical process, such as numbers of trained staff. The effectiveness of the clinical process needs also to be measured by its adherence to best practice. It is of course also vital to examine the outcomes, both good and bad, in terms of clinical quality and patient experience.

External benchmarked indicators

There are a number of companies across the world which examine hospital data and compare outcomes. The most frequently quoted outcomes are mortality and length of stay. Length of stay is a proxy for quality since complications and poor quality inevitably extend length of stay. However, for both measures it is essential that the underlying clinical complexity and comorbidities are included so that the case mix from different institutions is comparable. This has resulted in the development of a range of indicators, such as the hospital standardised mortality ratio (HSMR), mortality from a bundle of 56 conditions with anticipated low mortality, etc. In the UK, two companies, Dr Foster and CHKS, have been leading on developing a benchmark service.

External analysis

In any organization there is a risk that the leaders agree with the good news about their organization and dispute any bad news. It is essential that there is a regular process of external independent comment and analysis of the organization. This comes from a large number of bodies, discussed below.

Trust-wide measures

Most trusts now have a range of measures which they monitor on a weekly or monthly basis. These are described below as dashboards. They are linked to those which are now mandatory and measured within the annual contract.

The main high level indicators for most trusts will include:

- Hospital-acquired infections and infection control
- Hospital standardised mortality ratio
- Timeliness of service delivery, e.g. percentage of patients achieving 4-h A&E wait, percentage achieving 18-week referral to treatment target and the list of times in which cancer patients must have received their care
- Measures of patient feedback such as patient surveys, complaints and litigation.

More recently specific measures of quality have been introduced. These are:

- **Infection control** – every trust in the UK counts every case of MRSA, and *Clostridium difficile* infection as well as other rarer hospital-acquired infections. Surgical site infections are counted. Bed sores which clearly predispose to infection are also counted. The trust is set a target of a maximum number of these infections.
- **Venous thromboembolism (VTE)** – hospitals now count the number of patients developing a pulmonary embolism or deep vein thrombosis in hospital as well as those admitted with these conditions. In addition, it is now mandatory to count the number of patients who have been risk-assessed at the time of admission for VTE so that all patients receive appropriate prophylaxis.
- **Global Trigger Tool** – the Global Trigger Tool comprises a set of questions that are used to interrogate a set of notes. In England this is used in two ways. Every month 10 randomly selected notes from those admitted are selected and interrogated. The questions in the tool identify elements of care where an error or failure in quality may have occurred. Each month the number of these is counted and the total is documented. The tool is also used to examine the notes of 50 consecutive deaths on a twice-yearly basis for the same purpose.
- **Never Events** – all trusts must identify any of a list of 'Never Events' where harm is directly caused through error. The core list of Never Events is wrong site surgery, retained instrument post-operation, wrong route administration of chemotherapy, misplaced nasogastric tube not detected prior to use, inpatient suicide using non-collapsible rails, escape from within secure mental health services by patients who are transferring prisoners, in-hospital maternal death from post-partum haemorrhage after elective Caesarean section, intravenous administration of mis-selected concentration of potassium chloride.
- **SUIs and incidents** – serious untoward incidents are a marker of quality problems and are documented and each one discussed in all NHS Boards. The total number of incidents is also a useful marker. Although it seems counter intuitive, the larger the number of incidents the safer is the hospital. The argument goes that staff notify an incident when they see something which breaches the threshold of what they feel is safe. The more they notify incidents, the lower their threshold for concern. The ratio of incidents with harm to total incidents should be very low.

Results from external inspections

The trust is in regular receipt of inspections and external reviews of the outcome data. These need to be brought into a unified whole for the Board to review. Important feedback from junior doctors is received following Deanery inspections and from the Postgraduate Medical Education Training Board survey. The juniors rotate between hospitals and are uniquely equipped to make comparisons between hospitals.

Feedback from patients

Feedback from patients comes from a number of sources:

- National patient survey
- Complaints and direct comments to the Patient Advisory and Liaison Service
- Litigation
- Local surveys conducted by different services
- Patient Reported Outcome Measures
- Patient focus groups
- Ward surveys using an electronic device to document standardized response to five standard questions.

Feedback from staff

Staff attitude and behaviour are intimately related to the quality of the service. Measures such as percentage of staff with appraisals and mandatory training reflect the level of management input into staff. Sickness, vacancy rate and turnover reflect staff contentedness. The results of the annual staff survey conducted by the NHS indicate their support for and confidence in the organization.

Financial performance

Whilst there is a risk that excessive focus on cost reduction may damage quality, more sophisticated analysis of the financial performance can give an indication of quality problems. High agency spend is a marker of problems recruiting and retaining staff. Failure of financial management in an area may be the result of a long length of stay owing to a high clinical complication rate.

Measures for each section of the organization

There seem to be powerful reasons for each section of the organization to measure quality indicators relevant to their own specific area of activity. This data can give assurance to the organization on the quality of what is provided. The data can also serve as the cornerstone of the evidence required by individual team members for their appraisal and revalidation. For instance, in emergency surgery, examples might include: patients not receiving emergency surgery within 24 hours of the decision to operate, unplanned re-operation within 48 hours (typically due to haemorrhage), unplanned operation within 28 days (typically other complications), unplanned admission to ITU, operations lasting >1 hour without a consultant present, night-time operations without a consultant present, emergency surgery length of stay and risk-adjusted mortality rate for the service.

Measuring the effectiveness of the clinical processes

We know for many common problems the five or six things which have to be done to maximize the chance of a cure. Despite this knowledge, audits frequently show that the majority of patients do not receive all the required elements of care. Tools such as care bundles provide a way to ensure and document that all elements are delivered every time. Presenting data on percentage of patients receiving all the elements is a recognized quality indicator and underpins the bonus scheme pay for performance in the USA.

Chapter

49

Patient feedback

In the commercial world, businesses that follow the mantra 'customer is king' are more successful. These collect feedback from customers and respond to meet their needs. In the public sector satisfying the voter is vital for government and they need to ensure health and other services are responsive to the needs of users.

National survey

The NHS conducts an annual survey of a subset of patients admitted to hospital each August. This provides feedback to the hospital and allows the government to compare the services provided by hospitals. Different sections of the survey focus on different aspects of care. For example, doctors are often criticized for failing to communicate properly with patients and failing to involve them in the decisions about their care.

Statutory groups

This is likely to change with the introduction of HealthWatch.

PROMS

Patient Reported Outcome Measures (PROMs) record the extent to which a patient feels better after an episode of care. BUPA have used these for a number of years. Patients fill in a quality of life questionnaire before and 3 months after a surgical procedure. The improvement can be compared by type of operation between surgeons. The NHS has introduced a similar approach for a limited range of common operations such as hip and knee replacement. Operations where there are well validated measures such as the Oxford hip and knee score lend themselves to this approach.

Patient forums and liaison committees

Different hospitals have different arrangements to receive feedback from the patient community. Most have some form of patient forum and for specific services such as maternity there is commonly a liaison committee.

Patient experience trackers

It would be good to know how every patient feels after every encounter with different parts of the organization. If we could measure this we could identify precisely which areas to improve. The patient experience tracker is a tablet PC device which asks the patient to answer a few simple standardized questions. The data can build up to give data on customer care in different wards or departments.

Mystery shoppers

Some organizations invite lay people to visit clinical areas and write reports, acting in the role of 'mystery shoppers'.

Patient stories

Patients are invited to tell a group of staff their story, focusing on the experiences they had as they journeyed through different parts of the hospital. Whilst only anecdotal, many staff find this a very powerful way to engage with the concerns of individual people and it can open people's eyes to problems they had not seen previously.

Suggestion cards

Some clinical areas have a box for suggestion cards and a board showing how previous suggestions from patients have been implemented.

360° Multi-source feedback

The multi-source feedback required under strengthened appraisal will invite feedback from patients on individual members of staff.

Talking to people

Just sit in the waiting room for 5 minutes and chat to some people waiting. Walk round the ward, talk to a few people and see what is getting them down.

Complaints

Complaints are the tip of the iceberg of negative feedback. It is important to welcome complaints, to respond quickly and sympathetically, and to try to make changes. However unjustified a complaint may seem, it reflects the perception of a very unhappy person. There will be more with similar concerns who have not bothered to complain and all will tell friends and neighbours their negative story about the organization.

Chapter

50

Managing staff

Healthcare is a people business. Around 65% of the budget of any healthcare provider is spent on staff salaries. Each organization employs a large number of people with a vast range of skills. As a senior doctor or manager you could not possibly step into the role of many of the people that you lead. When the chips are down 'it is the people who do it for you', as one of my past Board chairmen often told us. The difference between employing staff who are happy, motivated and give an extra 10% and staff who are demotivated, take time off work and when at work spend time grumbling in corridors, wasting 10% of their day, is the difference for the organization of a change in productivity of 20%. So it is really important to value your staff. There are a multitude of processes and procedures to attempt to make this happen.

Once you take on the line management of staff there are a number of key tasks in which you have to participate, and are responsible for ensuring happen, even if you are not empowered to take all the actions yourself. Each of these tasks is supported by a detailed procedure which will have been written by the human resources department in your organization. The procedure will be based on the current legal framework. Deviation from the procedure may render your actions outside this legal framework. It is essential that you take advice from your HR advisor especially if you are moving into conflict with your employee. There are five broad areas: getting a person started, managing normal working, special requests, dealing with problems, and measuring how good you and the organization are at managing staff.

Employing new staff to the organization and starting work

Writing the job description

This is the most important step. What do you actually want the person to do? The greater the thought and precision that goes into writing down the answer to this question in the job description, the greater the chance that you will select the person most capable of doing what you want. Most consultant medical staff job descriptions are surprisingly light on detail. Perhaps this is because of the politics of managing multiple views from individuals both inside the organization and externally, for example at the relevant Royal College, and partly caused by a desire to give an appointee freedom to develop their career in a direction of their choosing. There is a powerful argument that if you want a particular task done, it should be in the job description.

Writing the person specification

The person specification leads directly on from the job description. The specification defines the attributes the person must have to deliver what is in the job description. These attributes can be technical, e.g. competent accredited colonoscopist/ATLS trainer, or behavioural, e.g. ability to lead a team, excellent relations with patients. The person specification is then used during selection to test which candidates have the evidence to show they can match the desired attributes.

Recruitment of suitable candidates from which to select

Where is the pool of people who are likely to contain those suitable for the post? How do we communicate with this group of people and make the post sound sufficiently attractive that the good people apply? How do we make the process fair so that anyone who is interested has a chance to know about the opportunity and make an application? For a secretary, the answer may be an advert in the local paper. For a popular NHS post, suitable candidates may be regularly checking the NHS jobs website, and posting the information about the opportunity on this site may be sufficient. For posts where a unique skill set is required and potential candidates are unlikely to be thinking of changing job, it may be necessary first to employ a recruitment company to undertake a search to talk to people who may have the skills and see if they might be interested. Once you know you have a potential field of candidates you can then advertise in the most suitable place. This procedure is commonly followed for chief executive posts.

Selecting the right candidate

If you have thought through the job description and person specification properly, it should be straightforward to look at the CV and statement from the candidate explaining their suitability for the post to eliminate candidates who do not have the experience or present written evidence to meet the person specification criteria. This will lead to a shortlist.

Most appointment processes use an interview, and on some occasions other techniques such as psychometric analysis, assessment centres and work simulation are used in trying to define the best candidate.

The interview is a structured process where all candidates are asked questions on the same topics. These should relate to the job specification. The golden rule is that past performance is the best predictor of future performance. Thus it is better to ask what a person did in a past situation, since this allows you to infer what would happen if the individual faced a similar situation again. This is better than a 'what would you do if' question, which allows the candidate to imagine their actions, which may not be close to what they actually do. A typical interview should cover the technical requirements of the post, an understanding of whether the person has potential to grow and develop the role and an understanding of whether the person has the right attitudes to fit into the organization.

The mantra in some industries is 'select for attitude and train for skill'. This is a very successful strategy. Problems arise more frequently with attitude problems and it is very hard, if not impossible, to change a person's attitude. It is important, however, not to translate an appreciation of the importance of attitude into cultural bias or nepotism.

Other methods used in selection have specific advantages. You need to use whatever combination of methods allows you to test for the characteristics required in the job specification. If you have asked for a good telephone manner in a secretary it would be wise to have a work assessment where all shortlisted candidates have a work test where they receive a standard phone call and are graded on their politeness and efficiency at dealing with the call. In the commercial world some executives are faced with a pile of correspondence to sort and action in a short period of time. In medical appointments it is surprising that we rarely use a work assessment.

Psychometric analyses have been used extensively in business to support the selection of a candidate. These tests are expensive and evaluate the personality and attitudes of candidates. The objective is often to see which candidate is most complementary to existing members of the team.

Statutory checks

Healthcare is highly regulated and every category of employee has to satisfy a number of categories of statutory requirement. For example, in the case of a consultant, GMC registration, name on the specialty register or completion of specialist training within 6 months of interview and criminal record bureau (CRB) check are mandatory.

Problems in recruitment and selection

Many problems arise if unsuccessful individuals feel they have not had a fair chance to apply, have been treated unfairly, or there has been bias or prejudice. This might occur if a post has not been advertised, if the job description has been clearly written with one candidate in mind, if arrangements for discussion about the job before interview have been skewed in favour of one candidate, if the interview panel is perceived to comprise a biased group, if there is any evidence in the process that past personality clashes have been brought into the decision-making process by third parties, or if there is any question of race, disability or gender discrimination. It is good practice to ensure that there are records of the selection process and the interview, and to ask all candidates at the end of the interview if they feel they have been treated fairly, in case unsuccessful candidates subsequently wish to appeal.

Agreeing terms and conditions

Within the NHS this has been relatively straightforward since NHS employees normally enjoy nationally agreed terms and conditions. In other countries it is common for there to be a protracted discussion between the successful candidate and the employer before terms are agreed. Even in the NHS there are special arrangements for removal expenses, etc. and each employer will have a policy. If you are applying for and are offered a job where you feel you have specific contractual requirements, it is wise to discuss these with the representative of the employer between being offered the job and accepting. This allows the employer to offer the post to another candidate if you cannot agree. You will gain a very bad reputation, which may travel with you, if, having accepted the post, you then find you cannot take it up.

Recruitment incentives

In some circumstances where a post has been very hard to fill the employer may resort to a financial incentive to encourage applicants. This may seem a good strategy. However, it can lead to a spiral of wage inflation. If there is a finite pool of prospective employees, every other employer finds themselves obliged to match the recruitment premium.

Induction

Every organization in the NHS has an organization induction programme and a local service induction. Induction is where essential information to allow the person to do the job is communicated. Organization-wide induction covers essential rules, mandatory training and house-keeping issues such as who does what, where and when. Local induction is a more detailed version for the local department. It should allow the new employee to know about the protocols and procedures and how to ask for help, as well as basic introductions and timetables.

Managing normal working

Setting objectives

Every year every employee should be set objectives. The idea is that after a year a person should have learnt to do what they do better, and this should create some capacity to take on some new activity. Ideally, this activity should provide an interesting challenge for the individual as well as adding value to the organization. Good objectives should be 'SMART': specific, measurable, achievable, realistic and time-limited. In other words, it should be clear to everyone what the person will do, by when and how it will be measured. The objectives need to be within the control of the individual. Commonly, the objectives require the individual to gain some new skills and so they may be linked to their personal development plan. For example, a secretary may require training if his or her objectives are to start to take minutes of meetings or a consultant may need training if he or she is to become an appraiser.

Job planning

It is very helpful for every member of staff to understand what they have to do at different times in the week. Everyone needs some form of timetable. For senior medical staff this has taken on considerable complexity as different aspects have become enshrined in the National Terms and Conditions. For junior staff the timetable has become complicated by the competing requirements of service and training, and the European Working Time Directive. At the centre is the issue that medical staff are given a great deal of discretion in deciding their work patterns. This allows flexibility to respond to clinical need and encourages a broad range of very valuable contributions, but creates difficulty in documenting activity and demonstrating value for money.

The standard new contract job plan for NHS consultants comprises 10 programmed activities (PAs) each week. These have an average duration of 4 hours. Consultants are obliged to offer 7.5 PAs for direct clinical care which is not exclusively patient, sample or image facing activities but can include related clinical administration and meetings. They are allowed 2.5 PAs each week for supporting professional activities. There is a broad definition of what is allowed. The job planning process is a negotiation between employer and consultant to map out each year the pattern of these different activities, how they relate to the separately remunerated on-call activities and whether the employer is asking for additional PAs which may require additional payment.

All public sector workers are obliged to adhere to the European Working Time Directive. This is health and safety legislation that limits the maximum hours worked in a week to 48, limits the duration of work periods and requires appropriate meal and rest breaks.

Managing the day-to-day work

Good departments know in advance what they are going to do in the week ahead, have a plan in place, monitor how they are doing and have arrangements to escalate to second line plans if there is a surge in the work or one of a number of relatively predictable problems such as sickness occurs.

Maintaining strong day-to-day/week-to-week communications

In good departments all the staff, from consultant to the most junior receptionist, know what is happening and are committed and motivated to working as a team to get through the work. This relies on regular meetings and good communication. If all the staff understand the problems they are more likely to find solutions. In my experience, departments that have a short meeting of all staff every week rarely have problems. Departments where people never meet often get into trouble.

Appraisal

Most people like to know how they are doing. Most people work hard and so appraisal should be a positive experience. Normal appraisal will look at the quality of the person's work, discuss problems such as complaints or incidents, discuss how the person is finding the practicalities of the role (including time-keeping and any absenteeism), review the objectives and discuss how the required continuous professional development (CPD) was achieved. The discussion is likely to culminate in a written statement praising the good things and identifying one or two things to work on over the forthcoming year. In some organizations the objectives have a scoring system and this is calculated to feed into a reward or bonus scheme.

In the medical world in the UK, appraisals have become codified and driven forward by the Department of Health and the GMC as a means not only to evaluate how well a local employer feels an individual is performing, but also to ensure that the individual is meeting the standards expected from a fitness to practise perspective.

Staff development

Staff training falls into a number of types. Some staff, such as medical staff, need regular training to keep up to date with the knowledge and skills in their area of expertise. This is very important. Medicine is a highly technical subject where scientific knowledge as well as medication and the best operative techniques change frequently.

Training is also required to learn new protocols and systems for delivering care. For example, training staff in hand hygiene and central line care has made a substantial contribution to reducing hospital-acquired infections.

With the growing importance of patient feedback in quantifying the quality of patient care, many organizations are investing in training all medical, nursing and frontline staff in customer care.

Within a portfolio of CPD, those in leadership roles will need training in how the business runs and how to contribute to improving efficiency and productivity.

There are also a number of important areas of mandatory training.

Ensuring mandatory training

There is a fairly standard list of topics in which training is required for all new staff. Whilst those who rotate regularly between hospitals can find this irksome, there is logic. The training can save lives and, by documenting that training has been received by staff, the employer goes some way toward discharging its responsibility to provide a duty of care to the employees.

- Fire training is required to save staff and patients' lives
- Manual handling is important for those who move patients and lift boxes or heavy papers. Injury due to lifting is one of the commonest causes of time off work in the NHS
- Resuscitation training is important not only for frontline clinical teams but also to ensure that any member of staff can keep a person alive until the resuscitation team arrives
- Safeguarding children training should ensure that any member of staff can recognize a child who may be subject to abuse and knows how to access help from a paediatrician who can assess and manage the situation
- Safeguarding vulnerable adults is equally important although often more subtle. The elderly, physically and mentally handicapped are at particular risk of abuse by relatives, family, carers and staff. This needs recognition and referral to those capable of managing the situation
- Infection control plays a vital role in any healthcare organization. All new staff need to have strict instruction on the basic rules of 'bare below the elbows' hand hygiene and proper behaviour if they are ill, especially with diarrhoea, chicken pox, etc.
- Risk management is included in most organizations' list of mandatory training. Staff need to be encouraged to notify clinical incidents on the Datix or other incident recording systems. They need to understand that re-coding and investigating incidents are desirable as they are the only way that problems will come to light and be resolved. Staff need to understand the balance in the organization between an open reporting culture and a blame culture
- Customer care is a key requirement of any service industry and is part of the mandatory training of most organizations in healthcare
- Conflict resolution is included in some organizations' routine mandatory training in an attempt to nip in the bud difficulties in the work environment
- Other specific clinical issues are included in some organizations, such as pain management
- In local areas mandatory training may be required – for example, cardiotocograph reading for midwives, neonatal resuscitation in neonatal intensive care units.

Rewards

Why do people come to work? The work of Mintzberg and others identified a hierarchy of needs. The first objective of coming to work is to obtain what are termed the hygiene factors such as money to buy food and shelter. When these are satisfied people seek the social dimension of work and when this is satisfied they look to satisfy their higher needs such as a sense of self-worth and peer esteem. Rewards for additional effort need to play into this understanding. Rewards that make it clear to the person that they are very highly valued by their peers are most successful. Some NHS organizations have individual staff or team awards that give a modest prize but use a large ceremony to acknowledge an exceptional contribution.

Clinical excellence awards

The system of excellence awards for NHS consultants dates back to the 'merit awards' created at the inception of the NHS. In the current system there are nine levels of local award and four levels of national award, where the highest local level and lowest national level overlap. The levels create a ladder up which an individual can progress. The process is by application and the demonstration of an 'over and above expected' contribution in five domains: delivering the service, developing the service, management, research/innovation and teaching. Details can be obtained from the ACCEA website.

Managing the team

Failures commonly occur because of problems in managing the team. Keys to success are regular team meetings, ideally 30 minutes every week. Give an update on what is 'hot' or of problems coming up. Ensure everyone in the group has a chance to say what is bothering them. Tackle difficult problems head on, in an emotionally neutral and fair way. Ensure contentious issues such as holiday planning are dealt with openly and fairly a long time in advance. Remember that, in aggregate, the people in the room probably have more answers than you do.

Special requests

Managing home or off-site working

This is being requested more frequently and has many advantages for staff in reducing travel and for the employer, if 'hot-desking', allows reduction in office space allocation. However, home working needs special management to ensure productivity, achievement of objectives and value for money. The employee also has needs for work, socialization and interaction with their manager, which have to be met.

Sabbaticals, secondments and unpaid leave requests

Most trusts have a supportive policy to cover these requests. Employer agreement is required. It is vital that there is a written agreement to cover the arrangements when the individual returns to employment. This has to cover the date, any necessary re-training and eventualities if work circumstances change.

Locums: NHS, agency, non-PASA

Locums and temporary staff are unsatisfactory as they never gain the full local knowledge of the organization. On the other hand they offer a group of staff whose number can easily be flexed to suit demand. Locums can be employed at NHS rates and commonly existing staff are employed on this basis via the 'bank'. There are a number of agencies which supply locums at around a 25% premium. The government has a contract with a number of these agencies and going outside this list to the non-PASA agencies is usually more expensive and does not guarantee that the agencies have complied with all the Department of Health requirements.

Job planning

53

Job planning and appraisal and annual reviews all form part of the process of implemen-tation of the best and safest care to patients. Both are part of the revalidation system. Much of both appraisal and job planning overlap, but job planning differs from appraisal in that it involves the consultant and a medical manager plus or minus the consultant's clinical director. Its emphasis is on service delivery and patient care.

Job plans set out an individual's duties, responsibilities and objectives. The purpose of job planning is to review the range of work activities undertaken and to ensure that the workload is appropriately planned and rewarded. It must also take into consider-ation the trust's needs and ambitions. It is therefore based on a partnership approach between the consultant and his or her employer. It is an opportunity to ensure that the contribution of consultants is targeted at achieving both national and local priorities. It is stressed that job plans are not 'fixed in stone' and both parties should participate openly and actively consider alternative ways of working to enable service improvements within the job planning context. Job plans are prospective and allow any department to plan for its future needs.

The purpose of a job plan is to:

- Prioritize work and ensure a realistic workload
- Agree how a consultant can most effectively support the wider objectives of the service and meet the patients' needs
- Agree how the NHS can best support the consultant
- Provide and assist the consultant with appraisal and revalidation
- Agree a job within working time regulations
- Agree remuneration and a set number of programmed activities (PAs).

A job plan must incorporate job content, time and service commitments, and allow for any personal objectives that a doctor may have. It is therefore closely linked to the personal development plan that forms part of the appraisal process. The job plan sets out the main duties and responsibilities of a doctor's post and its service commit-ment. It should include everything in which a designated consultant is involved. It is important to specify those duties that an individual is doing as part of his or her job for the trust.

The weekly work is set out in PAs of 4 hours each and a full-time consultant is expected to work 10 PAs or 40 hours per week. Additional sessions can be added at the trust's discretion. Any programmed activity undertaken outside the hours of 7am to 7pm, Monday to Friday, is regarded as taking place in 'premium time'.

Clinical work

Clinical work is generally considered as 7.5 PAs in a normal contact although this will vary from individual to individual and trust to trust and, of course, for those with an academic contract. Direct clinical care includes outpatient activities, emergency attendance, operating sessions, including preoperative and postoperative care, ward rounds, telephone advice, multidisciplinary meetings about direct patient care, investigative, diagnostic or laboratory work and patient administration activities.

On-call commitments should be clearly laid out in the job plan. Under the new contract this is recognized in three ways: an availability supplement based on the number of colleagues on the rota and the typical nature of the response needed when called, PA allocation for predictable emergency work arising from on-call duties and occasionally, PA allocation for extensive unpredictable emergency work done whilst on-call.

Supporting professional activities

These are activities that underpin direct clinical care. They include all the other activities such as participation in training, CPD, teaching, audit, clinical governance, job planning/appraisal and personal administrative work. Programmed academic activities can also include such work as research, teaching and lecture preparation, assessment and examination of undergraduates and postgraduates, departmental seminars, journal clubs, national conferences, meetings and organization of courses.

Specific duties may be included, e.g. departmental rota organization, revalidation advisory duties, appraiser roles, additional job planning responsibilities as in advising and assisting career grade doctors, clinical governance responsibilities, infection control duties and hospital committee responsibilities.

Occasionally there are contentious issues in the job plan, such as the provision of a supporting PA for personal study or CPD which is left in the hands of the individual consultant. Increasingly, trusts are reviewing this PA in the job plan and for some individuals this needs clarification.

Additional responsibilities

This includes special responsibilities that are not undertaken by the generality of consultants in the employing organization and those which cannot be absorbed within the time that would normally be set aside for supporting professional activities. These are agreed between the consultant and the employing organization. Examples include being a medical director, clinical director, lead clinician, Caldicott Guardian, clinical audit lead, clinical governance lead, undergraduate dean, postgraduate dean, clinical tutor, regional education advisor, training programme director, college tutor, etc. Annual review looks at these duties, which often change.

External duties

This category includes other duties undertaken by a consultant that do not attract separate remuneration. These might include trade union duties, undertaking inspections for the Department of Health, undertaking assessments for the National Clinical Assessment Service, work for the Royal Colleges or the General Medical Council, acting on Advisory Appointment Committees, etc.

Additionally remunerated work

This includes a discussion about private practice duties and responsibilities, any category 2 or additionally remunerated work undertaken by a consultant. If a consultant undertakes private practice and wishes to remain eligible for pay progression or clinical excellence awards, the trust could request the consultant to work up to one extra paid PA.

Signing off and review

The job plan is signed off by the departmental head. An appropriate number of PAs must be agreed by both parties. Following the annual job plan review the clinical director or head of the department and the relevant NHS clinical manager will submit a report confirming whether the job plan commitments have been met and will jointly make decisions about career and pay progression of the consultant. Individuals have the right to appeal.

Appraisals

All consultant and career grade doctors must undertake a yearly appraisal. This is essential for the GMC revalidation process and an appraisee must provide evidence of compliance with the GMC attributes defined in the GMC booklet 'Good Medical Practice'. The documentary evidence must reflect all aspects of both one's NHS and private practice: clinical, education, research and management. For those who practise in many different places the main employer is responsible for the appraisal.

Every doctor must be allocated an appraiser who is trained in this skill and who will review and advise the appraisee about the appraisal process. Both the appraiser and the appraisee are responsible for the process and if there are discrepancies or problems with the process both are equally liable. However, the appraiser can only be held responsible for the information that is presented to him or her. If, for example, the appraisee says there are no complaints about him or her and there are many which come to light at a later stage, the responsibility lies solely with the appraisee. It is wise to keep a folder with all of the activity that is done as an ongoing process over the year as, for example, finding CPD forms and complaint letters at the last minute is stressful and often unrewarding.

Preparation

Appraisal documentation should be presented to the appraiser at least 1 week prior to the appraisal. The following questions need consideration by the appraisee:

- How good a doctor am I?
- How well do I perform?
- How up to date am I?
- How well do I work in a team?
- What resources and support do I need?
- How well am I meeting my service objectives?
- What are my development needs?

These questions form the basis of the appraisal.

The appraisal form consists of four major components and these are as follows.

Form 1 – background details

This is the information that identifies you individually and provides brief details of your career and professional status.

Form 2 – details of one's current medical activities

This allows you to describe your post(s) in the NHS and private sector and you are asked to provide what you do and where you practise.

Form 3 – record of reference documentation supporting the appraisal and report on development action in the past year

Four domains of reference documentation and information have been identified by the GMC, and these are assessed by both the appraiser and the appraisee together.

Knowledge, skills and performance

The knowledge component includes evidence of relevant undertakings of the past year's personal development plan, up-to-date relevant knowledge of all aspects of one's clinical practice, professional development with certification, and up-to-date knowledge of other medical undertakings such as teaching and management.

The skills component includes those required by law, those which are mandatory with the employer, relevant undertakings of the personal development plan, those which are a generic requirement of good clinical practice (e.g. communication, breaking bad news), those which are a requirement of a clinical specialty and educational, managerial and medical device skills.

The performance component demands evidence of performance in clinical practice. This includes completion of annual objectives, compliance with governmental targets, job planning and workload evidence. It also reviews performance in other spheres such as educational, supervisory, managerial and other roles held by the appraisee.

Safety and quality

This reviews safety, efficacy of care and patient experience. It includes patient safety initiatives, infection control, critical incident reporting and evidence that one's practise is compliant with NICE guidelines. Efficacy includes participation in the trust's governance programmes as well as audit activity, meetings reports, reviews from morbidity and mortality reports, outcome measures reports and patient feedback outcomes. Patient experience relates to feedback information, the management of any personal or departmental complaints, litigation, coroner's court activities, 'end-of-life' practice and patient feedback surveys.

Communication, partnership and teamwork

The key evidence in this section is provided from the outcome of multi-source feedback (MSF). This needs 3–5-yearly completion cycles for revalidation. It includes evidence of good record-keeping, consent, investigations into complaints and communication, any GMC issues, trust disciplinary procedures and documentation of any trust disputes in which the appraisee is involved.

Maintaining trust

This relates to appraisee probity and health as regards clinical practice. There needs to be supporting evidence relating to patient confidentiality, respect for patients in research projects, evidence of insurance for professional practice, a clean CRB report, a registry of gifts and other commercial sources of income, performances as a referee or medical expert and evidence of appropriate separation of one's NHS and private practice in terms of a job plan or equivalent.

Form 4 – summary of appraisal discussion with agreed action and personal development plan

This section aims to provide an agreed summary of the appraisal discussion based upon the previous documentation, and actions for the next year are agreed. The components from the above four domains are reviewed and agreed actions undertaken and signed for.

The personal development plan for the next year is introduced here. As many objectives for the next year as the appraisee wishes can be considered. For each objective it is important to consider 'what development needs I have, how will I address them and what additional resources do I require?' The dates for achievement and expected outcomes are set and, when completed, the appraisal is signed off by both parties.

360° multi-source appraisal

Part of the main appraisal documentation is the 3–5-yearly requirement of a 360° multi-source appraisal. Up to 15 colleagues (including nursing and administrative staff) from all aspects of the service in which you work can be asked to contribute to the process of self-assessment and -improvement. There are 12 components of care assessed by your colleagues and these are:

- Clinical assessment
- Patient management
- Reliability
- Professional development
- Teaching and training
- Verbal communication
- Empathy and respect
- Team player
- Leadership
- Probity and health
- Treating colleagues fairly and with respect
- Patient safety.

The appraiser assesses each component in relation to the appraisee and uses a 5-point scoring system comprising unacceptable, below average, good, outstanding, unable to comment. A comment box allows the appraiser to write freely on each component of the appraisal. All the information is then fed back to the appraisee for his or her personal review.

All the information from the appraisal is then sent to the trust appraisal representative who will review the appraisal with the medical director and the chief executive before passing on recommendations to the appraisee and the GMC.

Revalidation

55

Over the next few years, the General Medical Council (GMC) will be changing the way in which doctors within the UK are regulated to practise medicine. Revalidation is the process by which licensed doctors will demonstrate to the GMC that they remain up to date and fit to practise. The purpose of revalidation is to assure patients, employers and healthcare professionals that licensed doctors are practising to the appropriate professional standards.

How will it work?

Revalidation will be based on local systems of clinical governance and annual appraisal over a 5-year period. It will not involve a 'point in time' assessment of a doctor's knowledge and skills, but will be based on a continuing evaluation of their practice in the context of their everyday working environment. For most doctors, taking part in an annual appraisal will be nothing new. However, for the purposes of revalidation, it will be essential that these appraisals include an evaluation of performance against the professional standards set by the GMC and the Royal Colleges.

What will doctors need to do?

A key element in the revalidation process was that doctors would have to provide supporting information to demonstrate compliance with the 12 attributes set by the GMC in the 'Good Medical Practice Framework for Appraisal and Assessment' (Table 55.1). However, this framework and the specialty-specific frameworks proposed by the Royal Colleges for strengthened appraisals are currently under review following the GMC consultation and the need for a simplified process.

Doctors will have to maintain a portfolio of information drawn from their practice that will provide the basis for discussions at their annual appraisal. The evidence comes from continuing professional development (CPD), audits, outcomes, patient and colleague feedback to name a few.

Responsible officer

To revalidate a doctor, the GMC will require assurance that he or she is meeting the required standards and that there are no known concerns about his or her practice. This revalidation recommendation will come to the GMC via the local responsible officer. This is a new role created under the provisions of the Health and Social Care Act 2008. Although there will be some differences between England, Scotland, Wales and Northern Ireland, the responsible officer will generally be a senior doctor in a healthcare organization, such as the medical director. For GPs, the responsible officer is likely to be from the primary care

Table 55.1 GMC Good Medical Practice Framework for Appraisal and Assessment

Domains	Attributes
Knowledge, skills and performance	Maintain your professional performance
	Apply knowledge and experience to practice
	Keep clear, accurate and legible records
Safety and quality	Put into effect systems to protect patients and improve care
	Respond to risks to safety
	Protect patients and colleagues from any risk posed by your health
Communication, partnership and teamwork	Communicate effectively
	Work constructively with colleagues and delegate effectively
	Establish and maintain partnerships with patients
Maintaining trust	Show respect for patients
	Treat patients and colleagues fairly and without discrimination
	Act with honesty and integrity

organization on whose performer's list they are included. Every licensed doctor will be linked with a named responsible officer. To make a revalidation recommendation to the GMC, the responsible officer will rely on the outcome of a doctor's annual appraisals over the course of 5 years. The person conducting the appraisal, who will usually be from the doctor's own specialty, will have a crucial role in informing the responsible officer's recommendation. Once the responsible officer makes a recommendation, it will then be for the GMC to decide whether the doctor concerned should be revalidated. The GMC will need to be confident that the recommendations are robust, fair and consistently applied.

The way ahead

The GMC launched a major consultation on revalidation on 1 March 2010. Over a 3-month period the GMC consulted the medical profession, employers, patients and the public on how to create the right model for revalidation. As a result of the feedback the proposals for revalidation will change, although appraisal and robust clinical governance will remain the key foundations of the process. The overriding message from the consultation was that revalidation, while being the right way forward, must be simplified and streamlined and not place excessive burdens on doctors or employers.

The Secretary of State has committed to an additional 12 months of further piloting in England. This will provide an opportunity for further testing and information gathering about the practicalities, costs and benefits of the processes involved.

When will revalidation begin?

The UK Revalidation Programme Board, whose membership includes the four health departments, the BMA, the Academy of Medical Royal Colleges, the GMC and employer representatives, will oversee the implementation of revalidation. There will be no 'big bang' introduction, but instead a managed and targeted approach to the introduction of revalidation across the UK.

Revalidation will be rolled out only when local systems of appraisal and clinical governance are in place and sufficiently robust. Those organizations involved in early adopter initiatives are likely to be some of the first to introduce revalidation. The expectation is that this will begin in late 2012. The GMC will decide and announce when and where the first doctors will be revalidated once the components of revalidation have been tested and piloted, are embedded in local organizations and when it has assurance that the organizations are ready to support revalidation. Thereafter, revalidation will be rolled out over the following 5 years to all registered doctors holding a licence to practise.

What will happen to doctors who are not revalidated?

It is anticipated that the vast majority of doctors will have no difficulty meeting the standards of revalidation. For a small minority, revalidation may be more difficult and the responsible officer may not be in a position to make a positive recommendation to the GMC. If there are gaps in the supporting information provided by the doctor, the GMC may decide to defer revalidation to enable the doctor to collect the necessary information. If there are performance concerns, the recommendation could be deferred until such time as local clinical governance procedures, Deanery and College support procedures, National Clinical Assessment Service (NCAS) and GMC processes have been concluded.

The British Medical Association (BMA) statement of principles on revalidation

The BMA position statement of March 2010 set out the following principles:

- There must be a clear mechanism for dealing with conflicts of interest with responsible officers, including an appeals process with an independent scrutineer
- Remediation must be fully funded to ensure equality across branches of practice
- Medical Royal College standards for re-certification must be equitable, fair and proportionate
- Knowledge tests should form no part in assessing fitness to practise, whether as part of the GMC's generic standards for re-licensing or in college standards for re-certification; any multi-source feedback system must be validated
- The introduction of revalidation must be cost-effective and not put undue strain on the NHS
- Pilots must run independently and be fully evaluated, with the results published and fed into subsequent pilot stages
- There must be equality of opportunity to revalidate.

Summary

The introduction of medical revalidation across the UK represents the biggest change to the way doctors are regulated in the history of medical regulation. Successful completion of strengthened annual appraisal over the course of 5 years will provide the basis for doctors' revalidation. The GMC is committed to piloting and consulting on all aspects of revalidation before the process is launched.

Further reading

http://www.gmc-uk.org/doctors/revalidation
    (accessed 10 November 2010).

Managing poor performance

56

Staff need continual feedback on what they are doing well and how they can perform better. This is normal management. When particular poor performance occurs, specific or formal approaches are required.

Managing poor performance caused by conduct and capability

Conduct issues for doctors range from unacceptable behaviour such as rudeness, to threatening behaviour, to stealing, to criminal offences. Capability refers to evidence that the individual is not capable of delivering the safe, high quality care that is expected. An individual may fail in both areas and issues may overlap, leading to the phrase 'doctor in difficulty'.

National data suggest that at least 2% of doctors find themselves in some sort of difficulty in any one year. The size of this figure comes as a surprise to many and suggests that managing 'doctors in difficulty' has to be part of the normal business of any employing organization.

'Difficulty' manifests itself in a variety of ways. Behavioural issues such as lateness, rudeness, dishevelled appearance, inappropriate behaviour or smelling of alcohol may be noticed by colleagues or appear in patient complaints. Clinical failures present as poor outcomes in an audit, clinical incidents, complaints or litigation. A poor way for an issue to surface is via whispering in the corridor and car park conversations. This rumour-spreading approach does nothing to resolve a problem and only contributes to conflict and paranoia.

The way to deal with any suspected problem is to rely on facts, with prompt notification, investigation, documentation and then dealing with the problem. This can only be achieved by someone in a senior medical management position. At consultant interviews, when presented with a 'doctor in difficulty' scenario, it is common for the candidate to talk vaguely about discussing with senior colleagues and in the last resort telling the GMC. In practice the correct approach is immediately to inform the clinical director or medical director so that prompt and effective action can be taken.

The first step is an initial investigation. What happened? The essential element is the chronology, i.e. the precise sequence of all the relevant events with the times at which they occurred. It is also important to document why events occurred as this may identify system factors that contributed to the outcome.

If it does seem that an individual is having difficulties, it is helpful if the clinical/medical director can discuss any background issues such as domestic catastrophes or health problems with the individual. It is also normal to invite the individual to have an occupational health assessment. This provides a confidential opportunity for the individual to discuss issues.

The big divide in handling doctors in difficulty comes on the issue of whether the doctor has insight or is at least prepared to accept that other honest, reasonable people believe he/she has a problem. If a person has insight then they are on the same side as the organization in trying to sort out the problem. Far more commonly, the individual is in denial and suggestions that there is a problem merely stoke their paranoia. This leads to an adversarial position which can usually only be resolved by a formal procedure. One difficulty is that the professional advisers of the doctor are paid to fight the individual's case. This can reinforce the veracity of their position in the mind of the individual and prevent the development of insight.

Whatever the situation, it is important to use formal structures. Even if a formal investigation is not needed it is helpful to bring parties together to state to the individual, and then confirm in writing as a management instruction, precisely what behaviour is unacceptable and should not occur again.

All employing organizations will have a formal policy to cover conduct and capability. The principles are:

- An initial investigation is required to determine if there is a case for a formal investigation
- If there is, then the individual needs to be informed at a face-to-face meeting. They can be accompanied at the meeting by an appropriate representative or friend
- The formal investigation needs to be conducted within a specific time. It normally involves going over the chronology again, obtaining signed witness statements and ensuring that there are a number of witness statements for key events in the chronology
- If the problem is confirmed then results of the investigation as well as the arguments of the person involved will need to be presented to a panel. Witnesses will be expected to attend the investigation to give oral evidence. The panel will determine the outcome. This can vary from some further training or support through to a written warning, final written warning or dismissal. Commonly, advice would be taken from the National Clinical Assessment Service (NCAS) during the process.

The outcome of any formal hearing or management instruction would also need to be recorded in the individual's strengthened appraisal folder and, if serious enough to justify major sanction or dismissal, the GMC would be informed.

Suspension and limitation of practice

If a doctor behaves in a way that leads you to conclude that a patient they may see later today, tomorrow or next week might be at risk of harm, then the doctor must not see that patient. There are a number of ways to achieve this:

- Limitation of practice – if the adverse outcomes involve one particular procedure, can the doctor just stop that procedure until the investigation is complete?
- Supervision – can the individual be supervised for the activity under question? This might involve having a senior colleague work with him/her whenever a particular procedure or type of activity is required. Could the individual effectively work down a grade, i.e. a consultant act as a senior SpR until the investigation is complete? Where behavioural issues with patients have been alleged, could the individual be accompanied by a nurse chaperone for all clinical contacts?
- Suspension – sometimes it is difficult not to suspend an individual, particularly if the case is being investigated by the police or there is an influential external

recommendation that the individual cannot continue to work or the case is very high profile. In general it is better to avoid suspension. It is difficult to manage the re-entry at the end of the period of suspension and any external clinical assessment needs to be undertaken when the individual is immersed in regular day-to-day clinical activity. NHS bodies are required to report on the number of suspended doctors.

There has to be a balance between a number of positions: (1) the right of the doctor to be seen as innocent and not to have his/her reputation tarnished when a formal investigation has not been completed; (2) the importance of keeping a doctor working on some clinical activity to keep his or her confidence and skills up to date in the hope that they will be able later to return to some form of clinical practice; (3) giving confidence to the patients and the Board that there is no possibility that an incompetent doctor will be practising; (4) giving cover to the organization in the event that a presumed safe but 'under investigation' doctor then has a mishap and the organization is charged with not taking proper measures to protect the public; (5) treating all employees equally whether they be doctors, nurses or other staff. One category of staff cannot enjoy a different application of the disciplinary procedures of the organization.

Dismissal

In the final analysis the employer has the right to dismiss an employee once all the correct procedures have been followed. This applies to both consultants and junior doctors. The process includes the right of appeal. Although relatively unusual, a number of doctors are dismissed by their employer each year.

Managing other problems

57

Conflict

Commonly, things are not as simple as one person clearly having a problem. Departments can break down into separate factions with groups of consultants barely speaking to members of the opposite faction. This is an untenable situation. It is impossible for juniors and nurses to work in such a situation. However, longstanding institutionalized conflict can be very hard to resolve. The important thing is to recognize the problem. It may be possible to arrive at an agreement that there is a problem. It may be possible to use internal skills to go some way towards a secession of hostilities. Commonly, if the problem is longstanding and intractable, external professional facilitation is needed. Ultimately, it may be better if there is some turnover of staff.

Remedial training

Behaviour and attitude lie at the bottom of most of the problems exhibited by doctors in difficulty. Very few problems arise because people forget the dose of amoxicillin, but many occur because doctors are rude to those around them. It is said that people are like an onion, with their true personality at the centre and their behaviour on the outside layers. It is not possible to change personality, but we can change behaviour.

If an individual has insight it may be possible to use mentoring type skills to stimulate self-awareness and -improvement, particularly when supported by tools such as 360° multi-source feedback. However, by the time a person has reached the level of consultant, patterns of behaviour are more entrenched and change is more difficult. External professional help is usually needed. NCAS have studied a large number of doctors in difficulty and suggest that the older the doctor, the more difficult the individual finds it to acquire insight and to change.

Participating in any grievance, harassment and bullying or discrimination claim

All organizations will have detailed procedures covering these areas. They are taken extremely seriously by the NHS. In a grievance, the individual will believe that he or she has been selectively disadvantaged in the workplace as a result of the actions of others. In harassment and bullying the individual will feel that he or she has been demeaned by the words or actions of others, and in discrimination that he or she has been disadvantaged in the workplace on the basis of race, gender or sexual orientation.

These issues are dealt with by a detailed investigation, witness statements and a panel hearing. If the offences are proved, the perpetrator is likely to receive some form of disciplinary action. The victim will be supported.

In the event that the victim has lost their job and wins a successful claim at an external industrial tribunal, the organization can face a very large fine.

To ensure that employees have no case to make, especially when at the receiving end of management interventions, it is vital that every detail of the HR policies is followed.

Whistleblowing

Similarly, all NHS organizations encourage appropriate raising of concerns over patient safety and clinical quality. The individual who raises the concerns is protected by the whistleblowing policy. The individual must, however, follow the policy in terms of who to inform and who then to go to if they feel no action is taking place. For example, most trusts have a series of steps that must be followed before taking a concern to an organization outside the trust. For this reason, if for no other, it is vital that clinical concerns are documented through the established incident reporting database so that there is an audit trail of who raised what concern.

Occupational injury

A suspected occupational injury ranging from a needlestick injury or injured back to contracting a bloodborne virus infection needs to be addressed by the occupational health department. If you find yourself giving clinical advice or management to a healthcare employee with a suspected injury you should discuss this with occupational health so that you provide an appropriate opinion informed by facts which are within your area of expertise. It is usually wiser for the clinical management to be offered at an organization other than the one alleged to have caused the injury.

Industrial/employment tribunal

These are formal external hearings in an environment similar to a court of law. They can take a number of days. If invited to participate you should allow time in advance for preparation, ensure that you are well briefed and that you can attend for the required period.

Downsizing and redundancy

All industries have to 'downsize' during periods of financial difficulty. The NHS has been relatively spared for the first 60 years of its existence. Since 65% of the budget is spent on salaries, it is inevitable that there will need to be a reduction in head count if the income falls. The priority is always to try to protect existing staff wherever possible. This can be difficult in the NHS where there is often limited ability of one category of staff to cover the work of another. The first approaches used include: reduce agency and temporary staff; put a freeze on new appointments; reduce duplication of services; merge rotas; and reduce overtime or additional payment schemes.

As a last resort there has to be a process which selects posts to be made redundant. It is very important to remember that it is posts being selected for redundancy. Individual employees are not being targeted. Such posts have to close. When the people leave, the posts cannot be filled by new employees. The processes can involve voluntary redundancy (where staff are invited to be made redundant) or compulsory redundancy (where employees are told to leave). Best practice is to conduct service reviews to identify the minimum number of staff needed for any given service and then invite all staff to apply for the posts, recognizing that some of the existing staff will not be successful. It is helpful to have predetermined overt criteria that will be used in selecting successful staff, e.g. high quality commendation in appraisal, absence of complaints, etc. Other industries in trouble take a more draconian approach such as LIFO ('last in first out' – new recruits leave first – although there is a risk that this may be construed as age discrimination) or merely closing a whole unit or factory. In the NHS, redundancy within the national terms and conditions is expensive to the employer. Every so often the NHS has a scheme to encourage voluntary redundancy, which provides funding for a specific package for those accepting the deal.

Any arrangement for downsizing and redundancy is constrained by very strict rules, and there are stages where consultation with the unions is mandatory.

Hard-to-fill posts, recruitment and retention supplements

The mirror image can occur when an essential post has been advertised unsuccessfully a number of times and management wish to include some financial inducement either to retain existing staff or to provide an inducement for staff to join the organization. The problem with this approach is that there are a fixed number of hospitals and if there are too few available staff, the introduction of a financial inducement by one trust results in staff leaving other hospitals who then introduce an incentive and an upward wage spiral ensues. In practice it is better to find an alternative way to increase the pool of available staff.

58

Measuring how well we manage staff

Every doctor is a leader. In any group, medical staff are major contributors. Other members of staff take their cue from the way medical staff behave, what they say and what attitudes they communicate. The question for doctors is: through your leadership activities, do other members of staff feel energized and enthusiastic for work or the reverse, and how do you know?

Informal measures

Many people have a perception about the way their department works. Is yours a happy department? These views are often slanted by the perspective of who you ask. The boss may think all is well, while the workers are very unhappy.

Simple informal guides are: Do you hold a weekly meeting? Do all staff attend? Do people turn up on time for the meeting? In any given meeting does everyone say something? Does the leader talk for no more than 20% of the time? Have you thought of circulating a questionnaire at the end of the meeting to get feedback on your chairmanship skills? What is the atmosphere like at work? Is work conducted in a cheerful and purposeful way or do staff just gossip and chat rather than work, or perhaps there is an atmosphere of bullying and fear? What do the attendees at the staff meeting think?

Formal measures

Does your department achieve good staff management practices? What percentage of staff have had an appraisal? What percentage of staff have a personal development plan? What percentage are achieving their personal development? In other words, what is the hard evidence that the organization cares about individual members of staff?

What is your staff absenteeism rate? Do you interview those who report to you when they return from a period of sick leave and do you get a feeling that they are sick for genuine reasons only? Alternatively, do people just not turn up and no one really notices?

What is the staff turnover rate? Unhappy departments often have a high turnover of staff.

Can you recruit staff? When you go to find new staff does 'word on the street' make it hard to find good candidates? How many posts require a second advert?

Do you conduct exit interviews of all members of staff leaving the organization to understand why they are leaving and whether they had difficulties while working in the organization? It is said that people do not leave jobs – they leave their manager. To what extent is this true in your part of the organization?

What is the formal staff feedback? Do you have a quarterly or other regular staff survey? Do you sit down for at least 30 minutes for a pre-planned interview on a one-to-one basis with all those who report to you on at least a monthly basis? Do all those with managerial responsibility do this? How are your staff feeling? How can you support them through difficult times? If you do not know what to talk about, use the questions in the NHS staff survey.

The NHS national staff survey

The NHS conducts a survey of staff from across all sectors of the NHS on an annual basis to understand at a national level how well managed and supported staff feel. The questionnaire is sent to a randomly selected subset in every organization. The trusts are judged on the percentage of the questionnaires returned and on the responses.

The questions are in a number of domains. Work–life balance, training, learning and development, your job and organization, errors, near misses and accidents, violence, bullying and harassment, occupational health and safety, infection control and hygiene, health and wellbeing, and background details.

The questions ask the respondent to choose strongly disagree/disagree/neither agree nor disagree/agree/strongly agree to nearly 40 questions. Typical example questions in the 2010 survey were:

To what extent do you agree or disagree with the following statements about your opportunities at work?

a. There are opportunities for me to progress in my job
b. I am supported to keep up to date with developments in my field
c. I am encouraged to develop my own expertise
d. There is strong support for training in my area of work

To what extent do you agree or disagree with each of the following statements about working in the NHS?

a. I would recommend my trust as a place to work
b. If a friend or relative needed treatment, I would be happy with the standard of care provided by this trust

(http://www.nhsstaffsurveys.com/cms/index.php?page=survey-update, accessed 27 December 2010).

Personal measures

To know how well we manage staff we need upward feedback from those staff. Regular 360° or multi-source feedback is one way to achieve this. Obviously the questions used in the feedback need to be suitable to elicit the information required.

Emotional intelligence (EQ)

Emotional intelligence is the ability to connect with the emotions and motivations of other people. There are many who believe that EQ is more important than IQ in creating a high performing organization. Daniel Goleman, the pioneering author in this field, breaks emotional intelligence into five domains:

- Self-awareness – ability to understand one's moods and feelings, and their effect on others
- Self-regulation – the ability to manage one's own feelings

- Motivation – a passion and energy for the work the organization does
- Empathy – ability to tap into the emotional makeup of others
- Social skills – ability to manage networks and build rapport.

A good example of emotional intelligence in action is the speech in the Shakespeare play *Julius Caesar* commencing 'Friends, Romans, countrymen'. After Caesar's murder, Mark Antony, one of Caesar's few supporters, addresses the celebrating crowd and within a few minutes turns their emotions from celebration to cries for revenge against the murderers. The equivalent skill in healthcare might be when a clinical director has to invite consultant colleagues to reduce their programmed activities and thus monthly pay.

Emotional intelligence is thought to increase with age. This supports the view that, whilst some individuals are clearly more gifted, it is possible to learn and to develop emotional intelligence.

Absenteeism

Absenteeism is a particular form of behavioural and managerial problem. Across the NHS 4–5% of staff are absent on any given day. This figure of one in 20 is greater than in other industries. Unsurprisingly, it makes clinical services harder to manage. It was always said that medical staff had a particularly low absenteeism rate. This seems to have changed, perhaps because of the changing nature of medical work with the breakdown of clinical teams and introduction of shifts, and also because greater efforts are now being made to count absent members of medical staff.

Absenteeism is mainly attributed to short-term and long-term sickness. Short-term sickness may relate to a genuine illness or to an episodic decision to call in sick on a particular day. Long-term sickness is usually genuine but in some cases enthusiasm to return to work can vary.

Managing absenteeism requires a number of simple things:

- A policy which is clear, available and understood by all staff
- A robust method of identifying and recording who is absent on each day or shift
- A set of arrangements to manage those taking a short-term sick break, usually involving a 'back to work' interview by the local manager
- A set of arrangements involving occupational health to manage and regularly monitor those on long-term sick leave
- Importantly, it is necessary that people actually enjoy and want to be at work.

High absenteeism is a measure of the laxness of the organization in managing sickness and provides a measure of the extent that the work environment and team spirit motivate staff to want to come to work and not take a day off.

Chapter

59

Managing stress

Stress is the adverse reaction people have to excessive pressures or other types of demand placed on them. There is a clear distinction between pressure, which can create a 'buzz' and be a motivating factor, and stress, which can occur when this pressure becomes excessive. It is inevitable that events both in personal and professional life will prove stressful. Moderate amounts of stress provide the driving force for humankind to function optimally. Undue stress, however, is eventually unsustainable and may in extreme situations result in mental or physical disintegration.

Work-related stress is a major cause of occupational ill health. The costs to society have been estimated by the Health and Safety Executive to be around £4 billion each year. Work-related stress has adverse effects on organizations in terms of:

- Employee commitment to work
- Staff performance and productivity
- Accidents caused by human error
- Staff turnover
- Attendance levels
- Staff recruitment and retention
- Organizational image and reputation.

Recognition

There is a delicate balance between the positive effects of 'pressure' helping one to rise to a specific challenge and the eventual inability to cope with constant, unremitting stressful situations. At the extreme of inability to cope lies suicide. Medicine has a markedly higher rate of suicide than other similar professional groups and within it the specialty of anaesthesia has one of the highest rates.

There is convincing evidence that prolonged periods of stress adversely affect health. Chronic stress causes heart disease, gastrointestinal disturbances, sleep disorders, headaches, irritability, anxiety, depression, loss of concentration and poor decision-making. Stress can also lead to behavioural disturbances such as aggressive behaviour, alcohol or drug abuse, eating disorders and social withdrawal.

Causes

Doctors are hard-working, high achievers who make difficult clinical decisions under pressure, undertake a series of professional exams and compete for positions in an increasingly difficult job market. This all occurs at a time in their lives when they are forming relationships, moving house, starting families or facing financial pressures from growing families. With the break-up of team structures and departments becoming larger, working environments may make these normal life stressors more difficult to cope with for many doctors. Shift systems have weakened traditional networks of support. The mess no longer exists in many hospitals, and colleagues head off before or after shifts like ships passing in the night. The following are common sources of stress:

- Demands – excessive workload, unpredictable workload, unsatisfactory work patterns, work environment
- Control – lack of control over pace of work or work patterns
- Support – lack of support by employers, superiors and colleagues, lack of constructive feedback
- Relationships – difficult interpersonal relationships, bullying, harassment and other unacceptable behaviours
- Roles – uncertainties or conflicts with respect to roles and responsibilities
- Change – lack of engagement and poor communication during organizational change
- Pressure – time, finances, examinations, delivery of contracts, maintaining high standards, achieving targets, attaining desired posts, private practice
- Litigation – worry of impending litigation following a complaint, mistake or negligence.

Management

Under the Health and Safety at Work Act 1974 employers have a general duty to ensure, so far as is reasonably practicable at work, the health of their employees. The Health and Safety Executive has designed management standards to help employers manage the causes of work-related stress. This includes the undertaking of a risk assessment, taking active steps to identify stress risk factors and putting in place control measures as necessary.

There is a broad range of ways to handle stress. For stress caused by overwork, organization, prioritization and delegation are required, as is taking regular breaks and asking for help from colleagues. For stress of a more emotional nature, it is helpful to discuss problems with friends and family and share problems with colleagues. For general stress, socializing with colleagues and friends and having time for hobbies outside medicine are important.

It is essential in stress management to preserve personal time and establish hobbies to act as a diversion to counteract the undesirable effects of stress. It is important to discuss stressors with friends, family and colleagues. Regular physical exercise, relaxation and possibly meditation can help to control stress. Fundamental skills for control are those of communication, assertiveness and time management.

Support

When difficulties do occur there are many ways of caring for the affected doctor. Often the most difficult step in dealing with stress is getting the affected person to admit that all is not well. There has to be acceptance that there is difficulty coping at home and at work and the next step involves admitting the problem to others. Informal counselling or mentoring is often a valuable method of gaining insight and may be all that is required to put matters right. However, when there is evidence of a severe stress reaction, professional help must be sought. At a local level, help could be sought through the doctor's GP or by referral to the occupational health service and, at national level, the National Counselling Service for Sick Doctors, BMA Stress Counselling Service for Doctors, Association of Anaesthetists' Sick Doctor Scheme provide voluntary and confidential services to stressed doctors.

Further reading

Health and Safety Executive www.hse.gov.uk/ stress (accessed 16 November 2010).

Association of Anaesthetists of Great Britain and Ireland (1997) *Stress in Anaesthetists*.

The sick doctor

60

Shriti Pattani

There is an increased rate of physical and psychological morbidity in doctors. The greatest impact of being a professional carer seems to be on mental health, with both minor and major psychiatric illness occurring. Many doctors are not registered with a GP and may not have local access to occupational health services although this is improving. The GMC guidance expects all doctors to be registered with a GP. There is still a tendency to self-treat or request treatment from a colleague, which creates isolation and potential difficulties if more intensive support/treatment is required.

Sickness absence among doctors is traditionally low compared to the national average. However, doctors are as likely to develop mental health problems and may be exposed to occupational stressors that predispose to increase mental ill health. Concerns over stigmatization and confidentiality remain barriers to early intervention and treatment. Other practical issues for doctors in training is accessing GPs in their area or developing a relationship with a primary care physician. Depression and substance misuse in particular are thought to be the cause of the established increase in rates of suicide in doctors.

Poor performance can be a symptom of underlying physical or mental health or other issues such as personal/family stress, career frustrations, financial problems, personality or behavioural issues, which may be related to knowledge, skills and communication or, in fact, because of environmental issues – for example, problems with workload, bullying and harassment.

Fitness to practise and obligations

The GMC's guidance 'Good Medical Practice' makes it obligatory for doctors to seek competent advice if they are concerned about their own health. Paragraph 79 states: 'If you know that you have, or think that you might have a serious condition that you could pass on to patients or if your judgement or performance could be affected by a condition or its treatment, you must consult a suitably qualified colleague. You must ask for and follow their advice about investigations, treatment and changes to your practice that they consider necessary. You must not rely on your own assessment of the risk you pose to patients.'

Part of revalidation requires a doctor to verify that they do not have any health issues that affect their ability to deliver safe care to patients and they must recognize and act on emerging health and wellbeing concerns.

Recognizing illness in yourself and your colleagues

Early warning signs may be subtle. However, the following early signs, as identified in the document 'Managing Trainees in Difficulty', can be useful in recognizing illness:

- The 'disappearing act' – not answering bleeps, disappearing between clinic and ward, lateness, frequent sick leave
- Low work rate – slowness in completing procedures, clerking patients, dictating letters, making decisions; arriving early, leaving late and still not achieving a reasonable workload
- 'Ward rage' – bursts of temper, shouting matches, real or imagined slights
- Rigidity – poor tolerance of ambiguity, inability to compromise, difficulty prioritizing, inappropriate whistleblowing
- 'Bypass syndrome' – junior colleagues find ways to avoid seeking the senior doctor's opinion or help
- Career problems – difficulty with exams, uncertainty about career choice, disillusionment with medicine
- Insight failure – rejection of constructive criticism, defensiveness, counter-challenge.

Process for accessing help

If you become unwell, access either a GP or your occupational health department. Avoid asking colleagues to prescribe and do not self-prescribe. If a colleague appears unwell, encourage them to seek help through the primary care/occupational health channel so that there is a physician to oversee their care. If a colleague refuses to seek help and you have significant concerns you may wish to alert their clinical supervisor in confidence. It would then be the responsibility of the supervisor to ensure that the doctor is monitored, referred to occupational health or advised to see their GP.

National Clinical Assessment Service (NCAS)

Doctors can be referred to this service by their employer, whether it be the NHS or the independent sector. NCAS takes referrals where there may be health issues or indeed other issues unrelated to health, which are affecting the doctor's performance/behaviour. The aim is to help managers and practitioners to understand, manage and prevent performance concerns. The outcome of the assessment is a report to the employer with the intention of helping doctors to resume their job unless there are irremediable factors that would prevent this (www.ncas.npsa.nhs.uk, accessed 15 August 2010).

Sources of support

Practitioner Health Programme (PHP)

PHP offer free, confidential support to doctors and dentists working or living within the London strategic health authority region. It is a self-referral service for doctors with any mental or addiction problem (at any level of severity) or physical health problem that affects performance. Colleagues, family and friends of practitioners with health concerns can also contact the service for advice.

(Telephone: 020 3049 4505; email: php.help@nhs.net (accessed 15 August 2010))

Sick Doctors Trust

This is an independent and confidential organization that provides early intervention and treatment for doctors and medical students suffering with any degree of dependence on drugs and alcohol. The helpline is open 24 hours per day throughout the year.

(Telephone: 0370 444 5163; email: help@sick-doctors-trust.co.uk (accessed 15 August 2010))

Doctors Support Network

A confidential anonymous support service run by trained volunteer doctors (doctors for doctors) (http://www.dsn.org.uk, accessed 15 August 2010).

Doctors Support Line

This is staffed by volunteer doctors who provide peer support for doctors and medical students in the UK (http://www.doctorssupportline.org, accessed 15 August 2010).

BMA Counselling Service (available 24 hours a day 7 days a week) and the Doctors Advisor Service

This is staffed by trained telephone counsellors who are members of the British Association for Counselling and Psychotherapy.

(Telephone: 0845 920 0169.)

MedNet Service

MedNet Service is a confidential self-referral service for doctors and dentists in London who are in need of emotional support, in career difficulties or having relationship problems at work. MedNet is staffed by medical consultants, and interventions are individually tailored in the context of a supportive relationship.

(Email: mednet@tavi-port.nhs.uk, accessed 15 August 2010.)

Samaritans

This is a 24-hour confidential service that is available to anyone living in the UK and Ireland. (Telephone: 0845 790 9090.)

Support packages

Royal Medical Benevolent Fund

This provides two levels of support.

Back-to-work support packages; for instance, helping with childcare, study costs and maintenance while re-training following mental or physical illness. Help with grants or interest-free loans to adapt home or vehicle (www.rmbf.org, accessed 15 August 2010; telephone: 020 8540 9194).

Support for returning to, changing or managing a medical career, a family and your own wellbeing (www.support4doctors.org, accessed 15 August 2010).

Access to Work

This aims to support people to remain in work. People are eligible if they have a disability or a health condition that is likely to last for 12 months or more. An application can be made for support if you are about to start work, starting a trial of work or are self-employed. The service can provide equipment, adaptation to premises, a support worker or costs towards transport (http://www.direct.gov.uk/en/DisabledPeople/Employmentsupport/WorkSchemesAndProgrammes/DG_4000347, accessed 15 August 2010).

References

General Medical Council. (2009). *Good Medical Practice*. London: GMC.

National Association of Clinical Tutors. (2008). *Managing Trainees in Difficulty: Practical Advice for Educational and Clinical Supervisors*. (www.nact.org.uk, accessed 15 August 2010).

Royal College of General Practitioners. (2009). *RCGP Guide to the Revalidation of General Practitioners*. London: RCGP.

Index